GETTING OFF

A WOMAN'S GUIDE TO MASTURBATION

# Getting Off

Jamye Waxman

Foreword by Betty A. Dodson

Illustrations by Molly Crabapple

SEAL PRESS

Getting Off
A Woman's Guide to Masturbation
Copyright © 2007 by Jamye Waxman
Illustrations © Molly Crabapple

Seal Press
A Member of the Perseus Books Group
1400 65th Street, Suite 250
Emeryville, CA 94608

ISBN-13: 978-1-58005-219-1
ISBN-10: 1-58005-219-3

Library of Congress Cataloging-in-Publication Data has been applied for.

Cover design by RCD
Interior design by Megan Cooney
Printed in the United States of America
Distributed by Publishers Group West

To all the me, myself, and I's

To all the me, myself, and I's

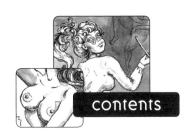

# contents

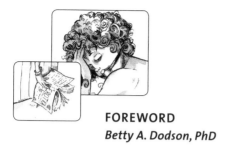

## FOREWORD
### *Betty A. Dodson, PhD*

ON THE VERY FRONT LINES of sex education today in America are the wise and wonderful people working in woman-owned sex stores across the country, and the women who bring sex toys to women at home parties. Both of these groups of teachers have the powerful and rare ability to come into direct contact with a cross-section of women and men and talk to them about how they can enhance their sexual pleasure.

The most incredible thing about sex education is that when an educator shares something new with a customer or client—a technique to try, a toy to include in sex play—oftentimes, that person then shares the knowledge with his or her partner. Sex education is easily passed along to others—even an inexpensive novelty item that will bring a few laughs in bed can open up new feelings and sensations; a goofy toy might encourage communication between a couple who've stopped talking about sex; a quality electric vibrator might kick off a few big, juicy orgasms for a postmenopausal woman who has given up on sexual satisfaction altogether.

Jamye Waxman has been an essential part of this army of sex educators. She has a master's degree in sex education, so she's quite knowledgeable—about the body, sexual relationships, sex toys, how they work, what they can do, and what women want. She's heard from the preorgasmic soccer mom living in New Jersey to the hottie twentysomething Wall Street broker who can't come with her boyfriend. I'm grateful to Jamye for sharing her insight with so many lucky people, especially during a time in our country when young people have no sex education at all. The abstinence-only-until-marriage message supported by our sex-fearing government has been a terrible failure, but at least we have intelligent women like Jamye to encourage awareness and impart new knowledge.

I'd like to say that we've come a long way since I began liberating masturbation back in the '60s. But when it comes to the acceptance of this basic sexual activity, I believe America has gone backward. I myself have spent a lifetime exploring different aspects of sexuality—starting with romantic loves, a monogamous marriage, divorce, and the swinging '60s, and then moving into the '70s dream of utopia through pot and universal love, consensual BD/SM play in the '80s, and twenty years of leading masturbation workshops. After all of this, I'm convinced that experience is the *best* teacher—and the next best teachers are the educators like Jamye Waxman, who enlighten, advise, amuse, encourage, and make sex and intimacy that much more fulfilling.

So start turning the pages of *Getting Off* and listen to all the ideas Jamye has to offer. Her love of sex shines through as she shares within these pages what she's learned. And then, after you do, consider sharing what you've learned with a friend or a partner. Because we need another million like Jamye to join together on the barricade against sexual ignorance. Make no mistake: Until we accept and honor masturbation as the foundation for all of human sexual activity, society will continue to be manipulated through shame and guilt by authoritarian religions and totalitarian governments. It's happening in America right now, and our best hope is to return pleasure-based power to the people by liberating masturbation once, and for all, and forever more.

*Betty A. Dodson, PhD*
Author of *Sex for One* and *Orgasms for Two*
www.bettydodson.com

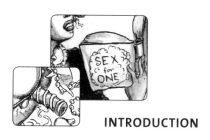

# INTRODUCTION

*MASTURBATION.* HOW CAN ONE simple word be so complex?

That's the million-dollar question, the one masturbators and would-be masturbators (as well as parents, churches, and teachers) have been asking themselves for what seems like forever. Let's face it, masturbation has been around as long as there has been someone who had something that felt good to stroke or to rub. Some still argue that masturbation is evil, more evil than the teacher who made you stay after school to scrape gum out from under the desks. Others believe that masturbation is healthy, like eating your fruits and steaming your vegetables.

*Getting Off* promotes the latter view, of course, and it's a book that's particularly focused on female masturbation. When I started researching the topic, I thought society as a whole had come a long way in terms of the overall acceptance of masturbation among women. But it turns out that acceptance has its limits. The truth is that we as a society are much more comfortable with guys pulling their chains than with women petting their kitties. Although as a feminist I'd like to believe otherwise, when it comes to celebrating female sexuality, we don't live in a society that values women the same way it does men. We still have a ways to go until masturbation is realized as a healthy, normal part of women's sexuality—which is why this book isn't only about how to masturbate. Most of you, if you masturbate, have a way you like to get it done. For those of you who don't, welcome, and I hope you find a way to masturbate that works for you. But for all of us, regardless of our experiences to date, this book is also a reminder of the struggle to accept and make peace with masturbation as an important piece of the sexual equation.

Most of us aren't taught how to masturbate; we figure that out on our own. What we are taught is how we're supposed to feel about doing it, and what other people feel about us, or anyone else, doing it. It's one of those things that we just don't talk about with others. I've noticed that lots of women would still rather talk about their last sexual encounter, or their upcoming date, than discuss the ways in which they can satisfy, or have satisfied, themselves. For every proud proclaimer of solitary sex there's another one who offers a disclaimer like, "I was desperate, bored, or too tired for intercourse." We need to stop thinking of masturbation as an excuse for not having partnersex, or a backup plan in case our partners fail. We need to remember that masturbation is the safest, most uncomplicated, and most easily satisfying form of sex.

I didn't come out of the womb tickling my clitty, and I haven't always been a one-woman sex machine. Ever since I became a strokette, however, I've enjoyed my sexual self so much more. I didn't discover the benefits of masturbation until I was twenty-one years old; I was already sexually active, and I didn't love my body, or myself, in the ways I should have. It amazes me to this day how I never cared about taking care of myself, or even making sure I came during sex (at least every once in a while). I was so busy wanting to touch everybody else and being the best sex partner I could be that I never focused on my own pleasure. Of course, life is a continual experience, and if I had not been where I once was, who knows where I'd be now. But I'm happy that I have no one to thank for my first orgasm but myself.

Before that first self-love Saturday night in the fall of 1996, I never even knew if I'd had an orgasm. I just assumed that I must have. (I *was* having partnersex, after all.) I figured that orgasms must not be as amazing as everyone else made them out to be. How could they be if I wasn't even feeling them, or knowing the difference? What I later discovered, after that first Big O, was that not knowing if I'd had one actually meant I never had.

My foray into masturbation started in my mailbox, when I found a sex toy catalog among my bills and other mail. I hadn't ordered the catalog myself (the former tenant had), so I took it as a sign from a higher being and quickly and eagerly flipped through its pages. I'd only recently heard something positive about a vibrator on *The Howard Stern Show*, of all places. While Howard touted the benefits of his wife's new vibrational best friend, I decided I needed a new toy for myself. The only problem was, I didn't know where to buy one. I was in living in Ohio at the time and the only places I knew were out in the middle of nowhere, the kind packed full of truckers and twenty-five-cent peep shows. This was before people actually shopped online, and long before the growth spurt of boutique sex shops.

That catalog became my one-way ticket to O-ville, and I couldn't wait to hop on that train. I turned its pages with unabashed curiosity and burning desire. My choice was the somewhat plain but reliable and, more important, inexpensive Slimline vibe. It came with two batteries, plus its own hard plastic carrying case. It arrived three days later, wrapped in discreet brown paper bag packaging—the kind that you'd pack your lunch in. Within five minutes it was on and I wasn't sure what to do or where to put it. When it met my clitoris, I snapped, crackled, and popped in less time than it takes to make a bowl of cereal. When I came it was like nothing, and I mean *nuh-thing*, I'd ever experienced before. More so than when I got my period, learned to drive, or moved out of my parents' house, I remember thinking that I was finally a full-fledged adult. For the first time ever, I was 100 percent in control of my pleasure. What a life-changing moment!

A few years later, I was living in New York and working at Toys in Babeland (now Babeland), an upscale sex shop on the Lower East Side. For five years I watched different types of women walk through the door. Some of them were braving their own personal demons, afraid to shop for a sex toy or admit that they masturbated. Some of them walked through the door nervous and inhibited; others strolled in with confidence and determination. I talked with all types of women, orgasmic and anorgasmic ones, single and married, foreign and American, and one woman who was upset that her religion had prevented her from enjoying orgasms up to that point in her life. She figured she'd lost a good twenty years. I spoke with hundreds of nervous women, telling them that their sex lives wouldn't be the worse for wear if they learned to make themselves their number one priority. I watched as their faces lit up when I explained how to find the G-spot or how to choose a vibe. I shared my own personal story about my self-sex blossoming, and I reinforced in them the belief that a woman is never too old, or too young, to masturbate. I loved, and still love, sharing too much.

In 2004, I got a chance to work with Betty Dodson, author of *Liberating Masturbation* and *Sex for One*, when she sent out an email looking for women to talk about masturbation and demonstrate how we did it for a video she was making. I had never been recorded having any sort of sex on camera, and I could hear my mother's voice telling me that while it was okay to work in sexuality, having sex on camera crossed the line. Still, I felt that if I was going to help other women and continue to help myself, this was the opportunity of a lifetime. And so I found myself heading over to the godmother (and grandmother) of masturbation's apartment to let my pants down. It was one of those awe-inspiring moments, sitting in front of the woman responsible for so many other women's orgasms. It was so easy to masturbate for Betty, and as she sat across from me, she touched herself a little, too. Eventually I came for the camera in the middle of Betty Dodson's living room. And when Dodson's video *Orgasmic Women: 13 Selfloving Divas* came out, I was the first person who spoke, telling the world how much I love to masturbate.

It was during filming that I first thought about writing a contemporary guide to masturbation. It would not be—obviously—the only book of its kind out there (I mean, c'mon, it's sex and you can't reinvent the wheel), but I felt a strong pull to jump on the masturbation train and praise the goddess in all of us. But it would still be another few years, with a different twist and with the push of a dear friend, before my idea came to fruition.

What I love about this book is that it's not just a guidebook; it's also filled with the social, cultural, and historical perspectives on the *M* word. This book details the anatomical structure of your genitals and techniques you can use to get off. But it's also about toys you can use, and why phthalates aren't your friends (see chapter 3, "The Buzz," or chapter 4, "Self-Love and Sex Toys," to learn what a phthalate is). It also discusses masturbation and piercings and female genital mutilation, and which lubes you can use to make the task at hand go more smoothly. I talked with and interviewed women from all over the world (thank you, Internet!) who shared their deepest desires, personal stories, and helpful techniques. This book is a combination of my insights and theirs, and you will hear many of their voices throughout these pages.

Chapter 5, "Self-Fulfilling Fantasies," is one of my favorites, delving into women's fantasies and supplying the juicy details about how women help think themselves off. Since the brain is the most powerful sex organ, I get into the idea not only that the brain is made up of matter, but that the brain *matters* in all sexual experiences. Chapters 6, 7, and 8 ("The Stigma of Solo Sex," "The Good, the Bad, and the Ugly," and "The *M* Word," respectively) focus on the sociocultural aspects of masturbation. In these chapters I debunk masturbation myths, provide a brief history of (mainly) female masturbation, and offer some modern examples of how female masturbation has been portrayed in mainstream media outlets, including movies, TV, and magazines. Chapter 9, "Enticement," is your guide to masturbation, complete with books, websites, sex-positive resources, and more.

I enjoy learning, writing, and talking about sex. It's my favorite subject and my driving passion. I'm totally intrigued by the struggle we human beings go through to love ourselves without having to love and/or be sexual with anyone else. It's as if most of us go through some sort of deep social conditioning, the kind that tells us that relationships are our goal in life, and therefore nurturing a sense of self-love gets lost in the mix. Many of us are reared to believe it's not okay to adore and appreciate ourselves more than we adore or appreciate our lovers or life partners. Through interviews, random conversations, group gatherings, and emails I've gathered that masturbation is still seen as selfish, and even though more and more of us admit to being a part of Club Hand, we don't actually proudly display our membership cards the way we do our engagement rings or G-string underwear. Masturbation, as a legitimate sex act, has been hitting peaks (Betty Dodson's 1973 NOW conference appearance; Shere Hite's 1976 *Hite Report*) and valleys (the 1994 firing of Surgeon General Joycelyn Elders) as it continues to climb up the ladder of social acceptance.

So what can we do to continue the membership drive? Honestly, we don't have to tell everyone we meet that we masturbate. But when we have the opportunity to listen to a friend talk about her failing relationship, or her desire to spice up her sex life, it doesn't hurt to suggest masturbation. Maybe she does it, or maybe she will want nothing to do with it, but admitting we do it in the right circles and situations will only help more and more women understand that they can do it, too.

I know masturbation is a choice, and the only one who can choose to do it, or to not do it, is you. Odds are, if you're flipping through the pages of this book, you have at least thought about going there. I hope this book encourages you to find your way, explore new and pleasurable territory, and continue to use masturbation as a way to stay in touch with yourself throughout your lifetime. After all, you are the only one who gets to love yourself forever.

*Jamye Waxman*
Brooklyn, New York
May 2007

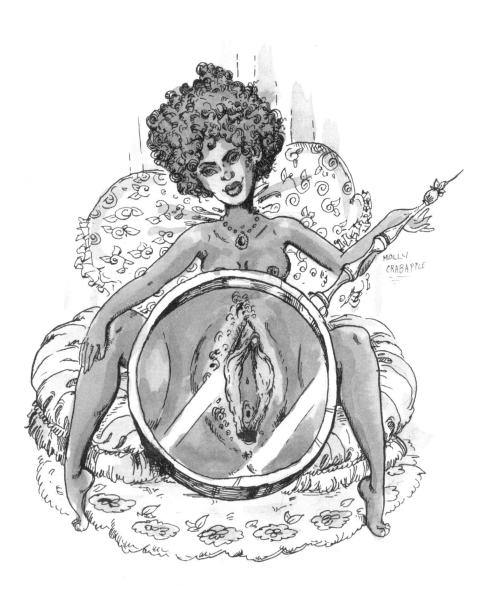

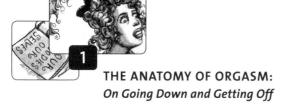

# 1

## THE ANATOMY OF ORGASM:
### *On Going Down and Getting Off*

FIDDLE, TWIDDLE, TUG, AND RUB. Flick, circle, tap, and tease. No matter what you do, or how you do it, when it's done to your genitals, it's called masturbation.

If you're a masturbator, raise your hand. If you're not, get thee to a private place, relax, remove those jeans or lift up that skirt, put your hand down your pants, and make nice with your pussy. Yes, that's right, start petting. Masturbation is like breakfast for your body, an essential component for a balanced and satisfied life. If you skip breakfast, you're more likely to be lethargic during the day and deprive yourself of essential vitamins. If you snub masturbation, you ignore the best way to get in touch with your own body, and you pass up a fantastic form of relaxation. Ultimately, both help you maintain a healthy body and, in the case of masturbation, a healthy sexuality. Plus, masturbation is a super-important way to figure out your own likes and dislikes when it comes to sexual stimulation. Of course, it's not cool to do it in inappropriate places, like at the family dinner table or during your English class, and it's totally wrong to impose intimate details of your handiwork upon others, unless they want to hear it, and unless you want to tell. Mostly, masturbation is all about feel-good sex—sex with the one person you have to love your whole life. Wherever you wind up doing it, getting off is a perfect way to relax, unwind, get in touch with yourself, and show yourself some much-needed one-on-one attention.

Now, in order to give yourself some proper loving, you need to know your own body, because until you do, you can't expect anybody else to know it for you.

 **GETTING TO KNOW YOUR BADASS SELF**

Have you ever sat with a mirror between your legs, examining the various parts of your pleasure anatomy? Do you know the words to identify the different bits and pieces, or have you just thought of the whole thing as your vagina for most of your life? How can you explain it all if you don't ever see it yourself? For most of us, figuring out what feels good often happens by accident. We may be riding our bicycles, doing pull-ups in gymnastics, or driving in a car when we notice that something about the way we're sitting, the strength of our muscles, or the vibration of the car is making our genitals tingle. This self-discovery can happen at any age, and does, but figuring out how to do it by choice, well, that can take years. This process of self-discovery where masturbation is concerned is quite different for guys. Stating the more or less obvious, a boy is born with a penis that he can grab, tug, and hold, which he does starting from infancy. With boys, what you see is what you get. With us, well, it's a tad more complicated.

If you've never taken a mirror to your genitals, you should do so immediately. Not only because you'll get to know yourself better, but also because a vulva, while not a super-sexy word, is super sexy. It's important to familiarize yourself with your clitoris, your labia (both the inner and the outer ones), your vagina, and your bum. It's important to understand your anatomy so that you're empowered and educated, and so you can see yourself as sexual and seductive. Our genitals are introverted by nature, and we need to find a way to bring out the beauty and pleasure that are inherently ours.

Let's start at the very beginning: All men and women are created equal. It doesn't matter if you're rich or poor, dark-skinned or light, heavy or thin; all of us have the same parts, just different styles. See, up until the eighth week of conception, all fetuses are on the fast track to becoming female. At eight weeks, certain hormones are released and others are blocked, which is when the Y chromosome traditionally makes its debut, determining maleness. Without the Y, there's no change, and a fetus stays on the path to a female existence.

When the Y chromosome exists and the male fetus develops, the result will be an infant who's got a penis; us female fetuses have vulvas. His bits and our bits are actually so similar it's crazy—they're just different in style. His shaft extends outward, while our lips fold inward. Our clits are tiny and sensitive, while his head is larger and still sensitive—but less sensitive than our clits. His testes hang under his genitals, while our ovaries float above. It's little details like these that make us different—but really, not that different. Still, because our genitals aren't out there for the world to see, or for us to grab, we don't always know how to handle what we've been given.

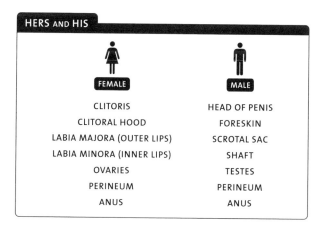

**HERS AND HIS**

FEMALE

CLITORIS
CLITORAL HOOD
LABIA MAJORA (OUTER LIPS)
LABIA MINORA (INNER LIPS)
OVARIES
PERINEUM
ANUS

MALE

HEAD OF PENIS
FORESKIN
SCROTAL SAC
SHAFT
TESTES
PERINEUM
ANUS

**BITS AND PIECES: ANATOMY OF A WOMAN**

Okay, great, we're built from the same parts as guys. Big deal. Now hand over the manual that explains how we function.

Bad news: There is no instruction manual. But at least today we have books, resources, and a cultural environment that's supportive of women's better understanding our own bodies and getting in touch with self-pleasure.

Prior to the 1960s, many women didn't know the proper names or places of their own genitals. The clitoris was often described as a tiny bump,[1] and not the intricate bundle of nervelicious joy that many of us now know it to be. Before psychiatrist and writer Mary Jane Sherfey wrote the most comprehensive article on female sexuality of her time,[2] women's genitals were often described in bunched-together terms, like *vagina* and *genitalia*, instead of as individual flaps, folds, and holes. In the 1970s, the artist, PhD, and sexologist Betty Dodson drew pictures of women's genitals, providing an aesthetic and artistic view of what was going on down below; in 1981, the Federation of Feminist Women's Health Centers published an anatomically comprehensive view of the clitoris, which was once thought of as the tiniest member of our genital structure. Turns out it's not: Instead, it's a large bundle of nerve fibers that not only sits at the top of your vagina, but also extends around your vaginal lips and works its way back into your urethral sponge. Without groundbreaking work like this, continued in recent years by Rebecca Chalker's 2000 book *The Clitoral Truth,* the clitoris, as well as the rest of our below-the-belly-button anatomy, might have stayed tucked away forever.

> *"It's generally believed that men's sexuality is more powerful and rewarding than women's is, but the big secret is that women and men have similar genital anatomy. The clitoris is as extensive as the penis; however, if you add women's innate ability to have multiple orgasms, then you'll understand that the clitoris is the real, and unacknowledged, powerhouse of all the sex organs."*
>
> —*Rebecca Chalker, author of* The Clitoral Truth[3]

## THE HOT SPOTS: FEMALE SEXUAL ANATOMY

There are a whole host of sensitive, enjoyable, pleasure-seeking nerve endings in all of our spots, and not just the places we know will get the job done. Take the time to get in touch with your body, all the way from the top of your head to the spaces between your toes. Now let's explore the hot spots!

### THE BREASTS

Those mushy, gushy, fleshy, firm, bouncy, bitsy, tender, toppling, pointed, dangling, suckly, large, medium, or small mounds of nipple, areola, and boob are highly erogenous for lots of women. The areola is the pinkish, mauve, and/or brownish ring of color that circles your nipple. Nipples can be small enough to simply brush, or large enough to pinch and pull; they are the antennae that can sometimes predict our levels of sexual arousal. All breasts contain mammary glands, used for providing milk to offspring, but boobs are also fun to grab whilst showing yourself some love. Lots of women like the addition of intense nipple stimulation through the use of nipple clamps during sexual activity. These clamps can range in form and function, from clothespins to specifically designed metal clips that are pinched on the nipples during arousal. Just a note: Nipple clamps do hurt, so if you're a beginner, try twisting your nipples with a finger or two while you masturbate before you move on to any other objects.

 The term *vulva* refers to the entire external package of female genitalia. Women often call their genitalia *vagina*, but that's not the right word for the whole package. In fact, it's like calling your foot a toe, or your hand a finger. Vaginas are a part of the cast, but not always the headliner, in our solo-sex show.

## THE MOUND (MONS VENERIS)

Also known as the mound of Venus, the pubic mound is the soft, fleshy patch of skin just above the vulva. It's slightly raised, and often described as padded because there's a cushion of fat right beneath it. Designed to protect the pubic bone (from things like the impact of intercourse), it gets covered with hair once you hit puberty. Your outer lips and your butt crack grow hair at this point, too.

 Gently massage the mons veneris by taking one hand and placing it on your mound an inch above where the outer lips meet. Move your fingertips in a circular motion, or press down toward your genitals. You'll feel the nerve endings getting stirred up. It's a great way to rattle your own cage, and it can really get you turned on.

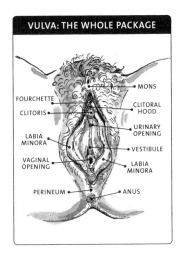

VULVA: THE WHOLE PACKAGE

MONS
FOURCHETTE
CLITORAL HOOD
CLITORIS
URINARY OPENING
LABIA MINORA
VESTIBULE
VAGINAL OPENING
LABIA MINORA
PERINEUM
ANUS

## THE OUTER LIPS (LABIA MAJORA)

The outer lips, or the external labia, are like a blanket, responsible for covering up our genitals. They're sometimes referred to as the "large lips," even though that's not always technically true, especially since some women's inner lips are way larger than their outer ones. The skin of the labia majora is the same skin that makes up men's scrotal sacs, meaning it's thicker and tougher in nature than the skin of our inner lips. And, like the scrotal sac, the outer lips have hair and are often the same color as the skin on the rest of the body.

## THE INNER LIPS (LABIA MINORA)

The hairless inner lips rest inside the protective shell of the outer ones. They are moist and soft, covered with mucous membrane, and positioned in such a way that they embrace the glans of the clitoris, the openings of both the urethra and vagina, and the paraurethral glands that lie on the sides of the urethral opening. The inner lips can vary in color from the palest of pinks to the deepest of browns, and they vary in length as well. They generally grow darker in color as they become engorged with blood. They can hang low, ride high, be barely there, or be wide and flared. They can hang outside the outer lips or stay tucked away behind them. They self-lubricate during arousal, and they come in lots of different styles and textures.

As a result of her once-negative views of her own extended inner lips, Betty Dodson, the grandmother of masturbation, likes to refer to individual vulva styles as "gothic," "baroque," "classical," "Danish modern," and "art deco." By pointing out the artistic beauty of every individual woman's composition, she's helped myriad women learn to love and appreciate the unique forms of their genitals.

## THE CLITORAL HOOD (PREPUCE)

This is the protective hood of flesh that covers your clitoral glans (head) and a portion of your clitoral shaft. The clitoral hood protects these parts the way a hooded sweatshirt protects your head. The hood develops as part of the inner lips, and it's the anatomical equivalent of a man's foreskin (for those guys who still have one), which is designed to cover the head of the penis.

Sometimes the clitoral hood is large and completely covers the glans; sometimes it's not quite that big. The hood might retract, or it might not. The point is, there is no right or wrong shape or size for the hood, or for any other part of your genitals, for that matter. And yes, women do pierce here, which isn't as painful as it is psychologically jarring.

 Use your hood when you masturbate. Press down on it to play with your shaft or pull it back and forth and rub the glans in between it. Or rub them together as a set. If you pull back the hood too quickly, you might overexpose the clitoris, and that can feel funny, in a not-so-ha-ha way.

## THE CLITORIS

No longer thought of as the immature predecessor to the vagina, the clitoris has officially been given a leading role when it comes to female pleasure. The only organ in the human body designed for feel-good fun, it contains about eight thousand nerve fibers, which means it has way more nerve endings than the penis

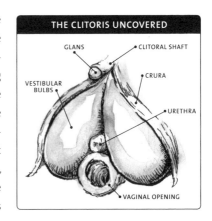

THE CLITORIS UNCOVERED

GLANS
CLITORAL SHAFT
CRURA
VESTIBULAR BULBS
URETHRA
VAGINAL OPENING

(the entire penis has about four thousand, in case you're keeping score). Taking a peek under the clitoral hood won't show you all its parts, though. You'll need to feel around to get the full effect. There are three basic parts to the clit: the glans, the shaft, and the legs.

### •••THE GLANS•••

Rebecca Chalker calls the glans, or the head of the clitoris, "the crown jewel of the clitoral system."[4] The glans is the most popular place on the playground, and the most visible portion of the clitoral structure. It looks like a tiny penis head, only without the hole, and it's super sensitive to touch, which is why it's got the protective hood.

### •••THE SHAFT•••

Spongy erectile tissue sounds like something you would use in the bath, but it's actually what the shaft of your clitoris is made of. The shaft, located underneath the clitoral hood and above and beyond the glans, connects the glans to the legs of the clitoris. It's totally tubular and generally longer than it is wide. It might remind you of the shaft on a penis, and, along with the glans (which looks like the head of a penis), the clitoris does indeed look like a smaller, more sensitive version of a guy's dick. In order to feel your shaft, rub on your hood and notice the spongy, cordlike structure. If you're at the beginning of getting turned on, you may feel your shaft engorge with blood. That's right: your very own erection.

### •••THE LEGS (CRURA)•••

The tubelike shaft is attached on one end to the glans, and on the other end to two clitoral legs called crura. These crura split from the shaft somewhere in the base of the mound, around the spot known as the front commissure, and then fall to the left and the right of the lips, urethra, and vagina. Picture, if you will, Thanksgiving dinner and the wishbone in the turkey, with one exception. Unlike that wishbone, you can't—and wouldn't want to—break the crura apart for good luck. In fact, you can't actually touch the crura, but they can help you feel even more sensation.

 More than meets the eye: The clitoris has a higher concentration of nerve endings than anywhere else in the body.

### THE VESTIBULAR BULBS (CLITORAL BULBS)

Lying directly under the outer lips, on both sides of our vagina, is a large wad of erectile tissue. Described as teardrop shaped, this corpus cavernosum erectile tissue (the same type of tissue found in the shaft of the penis) is a more substantial structure than the crura, even though the tissues connect, like the crura, at the shaft. You can feel these when you're totally turned on, because they become engorged with blood, meaning they grow in size and firm up the area around the vaginal opening.

 Try engorging the vestibular bulbs before going directly to the glans of your clitoris. It feels better to get aroused from the outside in than it does the other way around—especially since as we warm up, our bodies become more and more receptive to touch in places with higher concentrations of nerve endings, like the clitoris.

### THE FRONT COMMISSURE

This is the smooth surface at the bottom of the pubic mound where the top of the outer lips meets the clitoris. It's the area above the head of the clit where you'll find the clitoral shaft connecting with the outer lips. When you rub the front commissure you're actually making contact with the back portion of the visible shaft, and you can feel that sinewy shaft as you press around. And having more access to the shaft makes the front commissure a great place to connect with during masturbation.

## THE FRENULUM

On guys, this is the V shape on the underside of the penis where the head meets the shaft. On us ladies, it's also a V shape, and it's the place where the inner lips meet, right under the glans of our clitoris.

## THE FOURCHETTE (FRENULUM LABIORUM PUDENDI)

French for "little fork," the fourchette is the meeting place at the bottom of the inner lips. For some women, a light touch in these parts is enough to turn them on.

## THE URETHRA

This tube connects the bladder to the outside of the body; its primary function is elimination. But the urethra is also surrounded by spongy erectile tissue that's highly excitable. Its opening is a tiny hole located above the vaginal opening. You don't want to stick anything in there—that can lead to urinary tract infections and other unpleasant bacterial problems—but still, a lot of women like how it feels to touch around the urethra.

## THE URETHRAL SPONGE

This spongy erectile tissue contains teeny-weeny glands (similar to a man's prostate gland) that produce an alkaline fluid. All of the glands are collectively called the paraurethral glands, and they are the highly contested source of female ejaculation. Also referred to as the Skene's glands, they're located super close to the urethral opening.

"My roommate's ex-girlfriend can squirt and describes it as a feeling like you're almost going to pee your pants right before it happens. She says that the trick is just relaxing. And I just found out that one of my best friends is secretly a champion squirter! She says that there definitely has to be penetration involved, but that nothing can be inside when it's actually happening. I can't squirt and I'm pretty convinced that either you can squirt or you can't. I don't really feel like it's a learned technique."

—Lauren, age twenty-four

## G-SPOT: MYTH OR MIRACLE?

With the 1982 publication of *The G-Spot: And Other Discoveries About Human Sexuality,* by Alice Kahn Ladas, Beverly Whipple, and John D. Perry, the G-spot was pushed out of the body and into the limelight. Originally identified as the "corpus spongiosum"—the same tissue that surrounds a guy's urethra—it became known as the "Gräfenberg spot," or G-spot, after the German gynecologist Dr. Ernst Gräfenberg, who published an article in the *International Journal of Sexology* titled "The Role of Urethra in Female Orgasm" in 1950.[5] In it he claimed that there was no spot on a woman's body that could not be aroused, and made reference to the area that eventually became known as the G-spot. He called it "an erotic zone" that could be found on "the anterior wall of the vagina along the course of the urethra." Needless to say, Gräfenberg's report caused quite a stir, and, well, the rest is history.

When you're sexually excited, you can feel your urethral sponge (the G-spot is located there) by putting a finger or two inside your vagina and pressing toward your belly button. It's felt through the top wall of your vagina, and it's walnut-shelly in texture. The G-spot can feel really sensitive to touch and even make you feel like you're about to pee. Apply pressure when touching yourself there, since you have to go through a wall of muscle to get your "G" on, and never go into the urethra to find it. It's just too easy to introduce bacteria into the urethra, which can cause all sorts of unpleasantness.

## HITTING THE SPOT: G

HERE'S A STEP-BY-STEP GUIDE TO MAKING IT HAPPEN:

1. Go to the bathroom before you get started if you have any concern that you might have to pee.

2. Lie on your back, legs spread.

3. Get in the mood by touching your mound, your lips, and your clitoris.

**HOW TO HIT THE G-SPOT**

4. When you're gready (good + ready), slowly insert one or two fingers into your vagina, approximately one or two finger-bends inward.

5. Curve the fingers in a "Come here, big boy" motion, and gently hook the finger around the pubic bone—that means the tip of your finger should be pointing toward your belly button.

6. Feel for a zone, an area about the size of a dime or a quarter, with the lumpy, bumpy texture of a walnut shell.

7. Apply some pressure and stroke the area to increase the sensation.

8. Continue to stroke until it feels so good you can't help it anymore and you have to let go.

## THE VAGINA

In layperson's terms, the vagina is the birth canal—because, yes, that's the place where fetuses that have reached full-blown babyhood eventually enter the world (unless, of course, you have a C-section). It's also a highly erogenous zone, a sort of elastic tube that ends at the cervix, which in turn leads to the uterus. It expands when you're aroused, and the first third of the vagina is way more sensitive then the rest of the space.

### EXTRA CREDIT VAGINA INFORMATION

- The vagina is three to four inches long in its nonaroused state, and it can balloon to up to six or seven inches when aroused. That's why you can comfortably have intercourse with a penis (the average penis is five and a half inches) and give birth.
- Because the back part of the vagina is way less sensitive, you can surgically operate on the second two-thirds of the vagina without using any anesthetic. The real question is, why would you want to?

## THE PERINEUM

Affectionately dubbed the "taint," as in "'taint your ass, 'taint your pussy," the perineum is the smooth skin in between your anus and your vulva. There is also some dense erectile tissue down there which lies right under the perineum. Like other erectile tissue, it likes to be touched when it's gready (good and ready).

## THE ANUS

The anus is the most misunderstood sexual pathway because of its stigma of being a shithole. No longer 100 percent taboo, this equal opportunity orifice is another entryway through which to stimulate the G-spot and vagina. The wall between the butt and the pussy is super thin, and inserting something up your bum while you masturbate can be a fully satisfying experience, especially since there are a high concentration of sexual nerves clustered between these two places. Plus, the rectum has a lot of its own sensitive nerve endings that feel great when touched, and you can access them only through the butt. Your anus is a rather tight orifice, and therefore anything that goes up there can truly be felt to its fullest potential, which allows you to get the most out of these backdoor sensations.

**TIP** Anal penetration requires lots of lubrication and relaxation, along with a little bit of handiwork. That's because there are two anal sphincter muscles: one that we voluntarily control, and one that we have no control over. This second sphincter muscle requires a finger or toy to help it loosen up and let go, and since the butt doesn't self-lubricate, that means use lots of lube when you're heading upstream.

## THE PUBOCOCCYGEUS MUSCLE

If anyone's ever told you to practice your Kegel exercises, odds are you're familiar with your pelvic floor muscles. If you don't know about either these muscles or the exercises, read on. There are actually several layers of pelvic floor muscles, with the best known being the levator ani, or pubococcygeus muscle, also known as the PC muscle. The urethra, vagina, and anus all pass through the PC muscle. The PC muscle is a hammocklike muscle that stretches from the pubic bone to the tailbone. It not only helps stop you from peeing in your pants, but it also can help improve sex, help your orgasms become more intense, and make things easier during childbirth. Basically, if you want to have better orgasms when you masturbate, you need to learn to strengthen the PC muscle. Trust me, you'll be feeling it "O" so much more in no time.

## ONE AND TWO, AND ONE AND TWO: KEGEL EXERCISES

In order to properly clench and unclench your pubococcygeus muscle, you're going to have to learn where it is and how you find it. First, down with your undies, and get on the toilet. Next, start to pee. Stop, start again, and stop. Once you're sure you know what muscle you're using to control your bladder movement, don't stop and start anymore. It's not good for you to keep doing that, even if it's the best way to figure out just where this muscle is.

Okay, now you know how to find your PC muscle. Next you'll need to learn how to do Kegel exercises. These exercises will help keep your pelvic floor strong, so that you don't suffer from things like peeing when you laugh, uterine prolapse (when your uterus actually slides into your vaginal cavity), and loose muscles after pregnancy (how uterine prolapse often happens). And they definitely improve your sex life—both solo and with others!

Now that you know which muscles to clench and release, give it a try. Tighten and relax them over the course of a day. Start by trying to hold each clench for three seconds (make sure you're not tightening your ass muscles when you do this), and then release. If at first you find that you're clenching your ass muscles along with your PC muscle, don't sweat it. Just sit back on the toilet and concentrate on what muscles you really do use. If you continue to tighten your butt cheeks while you practice, what is generally happening is that you aren't training the proper muscles, and therefore aren't getting 100 percent out of the exercise. Take your time and start slow, really focusing your intention on the front portion of the PC muscle. We often involuntarily tighten our assholes anyway, and the truth is, we could use the practice of relaxing these muscles too, but when it comes to exercising your PC muscle, you want to make sure you're strengthening the places around your vagina. Whatever you do, don't stress. Time and practice will help you exercise that PC muscle correctly. You can always place a finger inside your vagina to feel yourself actually squeezing around it, or you can try a toy and watch as you clench around that. You'll even notice a tiny lift, which means you're doing it correctly. If you're a pro, you can do this until you reach ninety reps, doing three sets of thirty reps, of three counts each. It's like any other exercise: Once you start to train your muscles, you'll build up strength. If this is your first time trying to do this, see if you can do five reps of three seconds each. Even that might be more challenging than you think. Still, once you get the hang of it you'll stop making strange faces and you'll be able to do these any time of the day or night. Even if you can't hold for three-second intervals, just flexing and releasing the muscles is a great start.

---

### QUICKIES: A GUIDE TO KEGELING

1. Sit on the toilet and pee.
2. Stop peeing for a moment. Then start again.
3. Notice the muscles you use to stop and flow. Once you feel confident that you understand what you're doing, don't do the exercises on the toilet.
4. Hold your PC muscle in for a second, then relax. Hold; relax. Do this in three reps of thirty.
5. As you advance, hold and tighten for three seconds. Then five. Repeat the number of reps. Do this at least three days each week.

---

You can do these exercises daily, or a few times (three to four is recommended) a week, but it's important to just do them. Change things up every so often. Instead of three-second holds, you can do a number of shorter pumps, or do some slow and steady longer holds. What's so great about these exercises is that you can do them anytime, anywhere: at work, school, or home; on the subway, on the bus, or in a car. Practice when you're out with your family or eating dinner with friends. My favorite time to do them is when I masturbate, because it feels so damn good to have an orgasm while I'm tightening my PC muscle.

## FEMALE EJACULATE: TO SQUIRT OR NOT TO SQUIRT

Before getting too far into this section, I have to confess that it would be ethically wrong, at least in my world, to not mention that this isn't something all women want or need to do. Female ejaculation (also called squirting and gushing, terms that imply a certain action every time you ejaculate) is not likely to make your orgasms better, although they may look pretty cool; it's not something that will make you a better lover or a more desirable person. But female ejaculation has gotten a bad rap for such a long time that I think it's important that it not go ignored as if it doesn't even exist.

Female ejaculate can range in color, texture, and amount each and every time you make yourself squirt. In smaller amounts, it's often thicker and more pungent. It can be clear, cloudy, or yellowish in color. In larger amounts, it's generally unscented and has a crystal-clear, fresh-from-the-mountains look to it. In both cases, the fluid contains PSA (prostate-specific antigen) and PAP (prostatic acid phosphatase), two enzymes that are also produced by the prostate. Though women don't technically have a prostate, our paraurethral glands are as close as it gets, and have been referred to (and sometimes still are) as the female prostate.

There are also traces of other elements in female ejaculate, like urea and creatinine (also found in urine), but they're not around in heavy doses. The female prostate is still very hush-hush because, unlike a man's prostate, there isn't an actual organ to point to—so you may see "female prostate" in quotation marks. But we're all built of the same stuff, and the prostatic material in our bodies has to go somewhere. More commonly, this area will be referred to as the paraurethral glands.

Most women "ejaculate," even if it's just a dribble on the sheets during masturbation or intercourse. It doesn't have to hit you in the eye for it to be ejaculate. In fact, the wet spot on the sheets—that's what I'm talking about. It's not always about squirting, even if that's a sport lots of women compete in. There's an argument around where it all comes from, whether it's from the bladder or from the female prostate, but the truth is that unless you ejaculate in a medical lab with all the right equipment to monitor your every move, you don't and won't know—and it doesn't matter. The point is that female ejaculate is real, whether you do it, don't do it, or have no interest in it whatsoever.

If you do care, then the next question is obvious: How do you do it? First, similar to the way you go about finding your G-spot, lie on your back with your legs apart. Next, you'll want to have an orgasm before you even try to ejaculate. Once you have that first orgasm you won't be so preoccupied with having to get off, and then you can just enjoy the wet 'n' wild ride you're about to embark upon.

> "Female ejaculation didn't have any major effect on me, other than Wow, me too? Cool. What has since irritated me about female ejaculation isn't so much that it has become a trend of sorts in the porn industry and amongst lovers, but that women are putting pressure on themselves for their bodies to react a certain way. I'm all for exploration and experimentation, but I'm bothered that young women are on a quest to become ejaculators, especially if they think it's going to make them more attractive or a better lover. It's not. Guys just think it's hot."
>
> —Anonymous, age thirty-five

After your first orgasm, when you're less sensitive and ready for another go-round, you'll want to move your hand in, past your G-spot, to another area (on the same wall, toward the belly). Sometimes called the A-spot, sometimes called the AFE zone, this is an area that will increase your vaginal lubrication, and it's the spot where you'll want to focus, where you'll move your fingers forward and back or round and round. Eventually, you'll get the feeling that you have to pee. As with G-spot stimulation, pee before play so that you don't really have to go, or at least not very much. Then continue to rock and roll in this zone until you feel the need to let it out. At some point you'll want to start clenching your PC muscle and playing with your clit (if that's your thing). It may take a few tries before you feel like you might want or need to ejaculate, so remain calm, be patient, and remember, it's all good.

When the wait is over and you're eventually ready, you'll find that your body will push out your finger, or any other dildo or object you've decided to use to caress your cunt. Then *bam!* That's it—you'll ejaculate. Like I said, it's cool, it's a neat party trick, but it's not something you have to do, or even have to attempt to do. And if you do do it, it's not something you need to be embarrassed about, either. Basically, the fact that female ejaculation happens tells us that whether you're a do-be or a don't-be doesn't matter. What matters is that wet spots are perfectly normal!

 GET IN THE ZONE: THE AFE ZONE

The anterior fornix erogenous zone is located just past the G-spot. Shake hands with your G-spot and then move farther back, feeling along the top wall of the vagina until you hit a zone that feels a tad bit rougher than the surrounding areas. That's the A-spot, the place you want to engage to both/either enhance your orgasmic contractions and/or try to squirt. Touch it, rub it, love it—just do it a little lighter and gentler than you would with your G-spot, because it's a bit more sensitive.

> *"I've been lucky enough to have experienced ejaculation five or six times. It doesn't happen as often as I would like, and honestly, I haven't quite figured out exactly how to do it, but the first time it happened was one of the best experiences of my life! The feeling of the orgasm coming on was quite prolonged and when it came, it was much more powerful than usual. The first contraction was really strong and I could feel the squirting. Although it feels as if I'm actually shooting it, I think it looks like it's just dripping from the outside. After I experienced female ejaculation, I learned that I can have as much sexual pleasure as I am willing to give myself."*
>
> —Mink, age thirty-six

## THE CIRCLE OF "O"

For years, sex researchers and educators have been poking and prodding human subjects about how they get off. Heading the modern-day journey into sex research was Alfred Kinsey, who was in turn followed by William Masters and Virginia Johnson. And it was Masters and Johnson, a husband-and-wife team of sex therapists, who came up with the concept for what they termed the sexual response cycle (SRC). After watching thousands of men and women experience orgasms through masturbation and partner-sex, they coined the phrase "sexual response cycle" to describe the physiological stages necessary to get people aroused and to orgasm. They wrote about the SRC in their own literature, which was made available to both the general public and other sex researchers, and described the four stages of sexual response as excitement, plateau, orgasm, and resolution. They were the first therapists to actually diagram how people got turned on and how they eventually got off. This cycle majorly impacted and influenced the study of sex, sex therapy, and treatments for sexual dysfunction.

A few years later, with sex therapist Helen Singer Kaplan's addition of an important component known as desire, the sexual response cycle became even more widely accepted and used as the pattern to follow when someone wanted to learn to get off. It works like an exercise routine, and the components are pretty straightforward. First, you need the desire to get off, which is like motivation to go to the gym. Next you need excitement, the fundamental element of finding what turns you on—or the fact that now you're actually in the mood to work out because you've found the perfect swimsuit for next summer, and you want to make it look good. Then there's the plateau, the place where you've found the techniques that you like, and from there you keep touching yourself because it's taking you to a higher level—in gym terms, it's the regular routine that makes you feel good about getting back into shape. What we all work toward is the peak: the orgasm when it comes to getting off, or the burn you feel in a workout, where it feels so good, you now know why you started exercising in the first place. This can also be the point where you reach your limit and you need to let go. Last, there's the resolution, the rest period (or the stretch and recovery, in gym terms). See, sex is exercise, both physically and emotionally.

While it provides an easy-to-understand and accurate way to compartmentalize orgasms, the sexual response cycle is still flawed. The SRC assumes that men and women are similar in the erection section, and that we get off in all the same ways, which is so not true. In fact, sexologist Leonore Tiefer, a major critic of the Masters and Johnson model, has publicly criticized the SRC for not focusing much on pleasure or satisfaction, or other psychological or social attitudes that affect a woman's orgasmic potential.

More recently, other sex educators and researchers have found ways to diagram a woman's sexual response in terms of the emotional and psychological ways we get turned on. Focusing on the mind, and the ways we seduce ourselves, the sensations we use, and how we surrender our bodies to orgasm, these researchers remind us that orgasm is part technical and part emotional. It's about how we feel, what we believe, and what we like as individuals.

---

**THINKING SEX:**
**THE PSYCHOLOGICAL STEPS TO GETTING OFF**

Sex therapist David Reed came up with his own version of the Masters and Johnson sexual cycle when figuring out how men and women achieved orgasm. His version varies from the Masters and Johnson cycle because it focuses on the emotional components of arousal, not just the bare-bones basics for what is or isn't physiologically happening to our bodies.[6]

**SEDUCTION:** Dressing sexy. Setting the mood. Picking out the music. Exploring fantasies.

**SENSATION:** Fingers. Feathers. Bubble baths. Sex toys. Our minds.

**SURRENDER:** Focusing on sensations. Thinking ourselves off. Coming to the point where we can't hold back any longer.

**REFLECTION:** Listening to our bodies. Relaxing. Resting.

---

So, what's this got to do with you getting off by yourself? First of all, it's just a reminder that you are who you are, and that means you're different from anyone else out there. And even though we can categorize our sexuality by response cycles and their components, you are ultimately turned on by your own fantasies, desires, imagery; you might get excited by your own hands, a vibrator, your thoughts; you probably get off in myriad ways, and when you're done you relax, even if it's just for a second before you jump out of bed. So even though you might get off differently than everybody else, you will still go through a certain biological process that is similar to most other women's. But your emotional, psychological, and social components will never be exactly the same as anybody else's, and nobody can ever compartmentalize you, or your sexuality, into a tiny, perfect package.

## O, OH, AND OHHHHHH: THE INEQUALITY OF ORGASM

I don't want to focus on orgasm as the must-have in terms of achievement, because it's not like you have to come at the end of every masturbatory encounter. But since it's often the goal, it's important to take some time to understand the different types of orgasms you may experience. All orgasmic sensations are individual experiences, so there's no one way to have an orgasm and there are no definitive terms to categorize what you feel when doing so. But since we come from a society that likes to label everything, lots of the types of orgasms that have been categorized and labeled are listed on the next page. They should be treated as frames of reference for what you might encounter.

For starters, what is an orgasm? An orgasm is defined as a series of rhythmic muscular contractions of the female genitals combined with waves of intense pleasure, which is then followed by a release of physical and sexual tension. Orgasms are the result of a buildup of muscular tension, and a pooling of blood in certain erogenous zones that eventually finds its way out through this type of release. Most forward-thinking sex educators don't buy into the idea that an orgasm is achieved or experienced in any particular or set way. Some women can think themselves off without ever touching their bodies. Others need lots of attention paid to particular parts. Still others come at the touch of a button. No two experiences and no two orgasms are ever going to be exactly the same. Sometimes your orgasms will be full-body, out-of-mind experiences, while other times they'll be short, sweet, and over before you even begin to shiver and shake.

The most easy-to-understand orgasms, in terms of definition, are clitoral, vaginal, G-spot, and anal. Masturbation maven Dodson, in her book *Orgasms for Two,* describes nine different kinds of orgasms, including "tension," "relaxation," "combination (blended)," "pressure," "multiple," "fantasy," and "meltdown."[7] Sex educator and author Lou Paget adds "AFE zone," "U-spot," "breast/nipple," "mouth," and "anal" orgasms.[8] Barbara Carrellas, also an author and sex educator, describes orgasms that have nothing to do with touching yourself "down there" or "up here." Her "emotion-gasms" include "giggle-gasms," "anger-gasms," and "cry-gasms."[9] These orgasms are more about emotional release than genital sensation. Carrellas describes orgasm as "a release of energy rushing through the mental, spiritual, and emotional body, connecting us to spirit."[10] That might sound a bit woo-woo, but the truth is, for a lot of women it's more like *yahoo!* It's important to know that we can have any damn orgasm we want. Sex-life coach and artist Annie Sprinkle, who once had her own five-minute "megagasm," says that if you feel you're having an orgasm, then you are, regardless of any one definition of the term.[11]

Orgasms are meant to be fun; they are also a great way to relieve pain, both physically and emotionally, and they allow you to connect with your body on a much deeper, more spiritual level. Orgasms by yourself and for yourself are a great release and a means of rejuvenation. But they aren't the only thing to focus on when it comes to masturbation, or any other sexual act. Of course, in the end, we all want some type of orgasm. It's just good to know that you're not limited to the muscular-contraction kind.

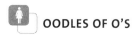 **OODLES OF O'S**

### CLITORAL

Clitoral orgasms happen because the clitoris is in some way rubbed, tugged, or touched to the point of no return.

> "I touch my clit the most because that's what is going to make me orgasm. Sometimes, if I get really into it, I'll grab my breast with the other hand. I'm visualizing a lot of other things in my mind, though."
>
> —Alison, age twenty-four

### VAGINAL/CERVICAL

Vaginal/cervical orgasms happen through penetration, and while Sigmund Freud declared them the cream of the crop, they are in no way the biggest, baddest, or best orgasms in the bunch. While some women are all about the vagina, only 30 percent of women actually orgasm from vaginal penetration alone.

### G-SPOT

A G-spot orgasm can occur without the aid of clitoral stimulation. Since the G-spot is not actually in the vagina, a G-spot orgasm is not a vaginal orgasm. For some women the sensation of having to urinate, which can come along with hitting the G-spot, makes this orgasm a tad more difficult to achieve.

### ANAL

An anal orgasm is brought on through anal stimulation by a finger, toy, penis, or tongue. A woman can stimulate her G-spot through the thin wall between the vagina and rectum. Adding clitoral stimulation can help, and some women can come just by stimulating the area around the rectum.

## FULL-BLOWN BOOBGASMS

Breast orgasms result from heavy petting of the breasts and nipples. Women with highly sensitive breasts can experience these types of orgasms. Add a little genital stimulation to the mix for added pleasure. Breastfeeding mothers can sometimes experience these types of orgasms as well.

## U-SPOT

U-spot orgasms are for women who like stimulating the urethra during masturbation. Since the urethra is surrounded by pleasure sources (the clitoris, the vagina, the pararurethral glands), this area can be a total turn-on for some. This is not about going inside the urethra, it's about stimulating the area around it.

## COMBINATION OR BLENDED

Combination orgasms are often referred to as "blended" orgasms. That means that you're not just coming through clitoral stimulation or vaginal stimulation. Instead, you're experiencing an orgasm that is the sum of these parts.

## TENSION

Tension orgasms come from direct, intense pressure in your pleasurable places. You're generally clenching and tightening your muscles a lot for these orgasms to occur. They're generally quick and easy and can be a result of having to find a secret, and fast, way to get off during childhood.

## RELAXATION

Relaxation orgasms tend to sneak up on you, coming from a place of deep meditation that's happening while you're being turned on. I like to think of them like a massage, where you're in a zone and all of a sudden the massage therapist hits the one spot that you weren't expecting him or her to touch that way and *bam*, you feel ecstasy.

## PRESSURE

Pressure orgasms are created by applying a certain type of friction to your genitals. Think of rocking back or forth, squeezing your legs together, or hanging out on the monkey bars. This is a hands-free orgasm.

> *"Once, when I was first learning to play bass, I was practicing this repetitive riff and sort of moving to the beat, and I got aroused and had an orgasm! It was strange, but perhaps kind of awesomely rock 'n' roll."*
>
> —Rivka, age twenty-seven

## MULTIPLE

Multiple orgasms happen again and again over a short period of time. They can be any type of orgasm, but they occur one after the other, generally without much rest in between.

## FANTASY

Fantasy orgasms are the kind that think you off, meaning that they result from your capacity to mentally get yourself going. Fantasy orgasms require mental stimulation to turn you on, and get you off.

### EMOTION-GASMS

Emotion-gasms are when "You allow your body to express its emotions without trying to stifle them," explains Barbara Carrellas.[12] They expand the definition of orgasm and occur in unstoppable bouts of laughter (the kind that leaves you gasping for breath, buckled over, clutching your tummy), or in loud moments of pain or hysterical moments of sorrow. Emotion-gasms are that extreme cleansing experience that allows you to come through on the other end. They're the kind of release that helps you to pick yourself up and move on. This orgasm does not rely or depend on genital stimulation.

Even though it's easy to get down to it, it's nice to allow yourself the time to build up to the dance of your choosing. Loosen up, let go, feel the beat, get into the groove, and then go to town on yourself. Don't always rush to orgasm just because you're getting off when no one else is around. You are the most important person in your life, a title that no one else can claim, and therefore appreciating your body and your mind is the hottest thing you can do for yourself.

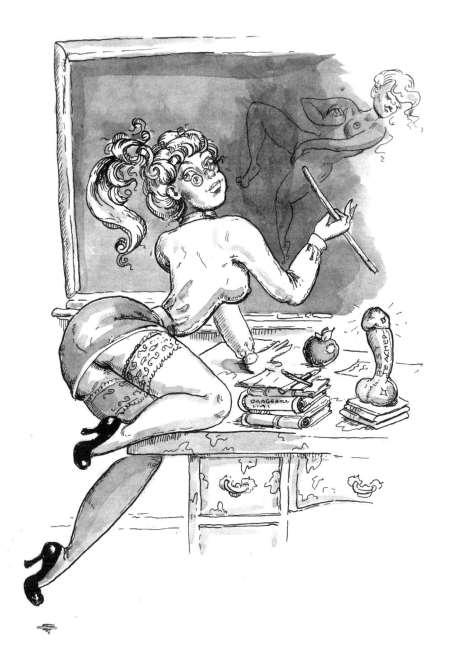

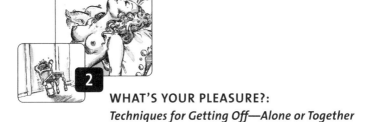

## 2

## WHAT'S YOUR PLEASURE?:
### *Techniques for Getting Off—Alone or Together*

THERE IS NO ONE WAY (or two ways, or three ways) to masturbate, and no one finger (or two fingers, or three fingers) to use to get the job done. The important thing to remember about self-pleasure is that you actually derive feel-great fun from doing whatever it is that works for you. No two women are built from the same standard mold. Penetration works for some gals and does nothing for others. You may like a little rub around the rectum, while another girl prefers to keep her back door sealed shut. And some of us need to ramp up our clits, while others prefer a good old-fashioned hand job. Whatever tugs, twists, or twiddles get you aroused, engorged, and on your way to release (if release is your goal), then that's what you need to do to get what you want out of the experience.

---

### XX AND XY DON'T HAVE SOLO XXX THE SAME WAY

Sex researchers William Masters and Virginia Johnson observed, and recorded, women masturbating for their sex studies (published in 1966). They concluded that no two women jilled off the exact same way. Whether it was in their timing, tempo, rhythm, or style, no two women danced to the exact same beat when it came to self-gratification. This was totally different from what Masters and Johnson had observed in men, who were less diverse and more general in their jacking-off ways.

---

Masturbation is no-pressure sex; it's sex done your way—by and for you. It doesn't matter how your boyfriend likes to get off and it doesn't matter how quick your girlfriend can come. When it comes to masturbation, Metallica says it best: "Nothing else matters." There's no pressure to perform, no pressure to get someone else off, no pressure to even finish the job, because the only person who matters during masturbation is (drumroll, please) you!

##  MOOD MAKERS

Since masturbation is all about you, there are things you can do to enhance your experience. In fact, the "room tone" can totally change the ambience and the attitude you have about getting off. Setting the mood is part of getting in the mood, so when you can, take the extra time to add additional oomph. A red room with silk sheets invites seduction; your parents' bedroom when they're out of town—or at least out of the house—adds an element of naughty. The front seat of the car with the stereo blasting the Divinyls' "I Touch Myself" can be a silly, fun way to get into your groove. Setting the mood is like making out. The more time you invest in the buildup, the more turned on you'll become, and the more likely you'll want to spend additional minutes making yourself feel good. Show yourself a whole lot of love before you ever get down to it, and you'll feel like a princess of pleasure.

### LIGHT THE WAY

Possibly the most important detail in creating an atmosphere is lighting. Bad lighting is horrific, while nice soft lighting is terrific. Think about it. If you're having partnersex with someone and you're a bit self-conscious about doing it under the glow of bright, energy-saving fluorescent bulbs, you're less into the experience, right? Dim lights or candles can make you feel like a million dollars, and they can add to the allure of seduction and romance. Instead of turning your bulbs up bright, keep a lamp nearby that emits a soft red or purple tint. You can buy a colored bulb in almost any hardware store or megachain, and it will noticeably affect the glow in the room. Plus, it will totally help you relax into the moment at hand. You can also do it in broad daylight to get in touch with your body in natural light.

> "Pink and golden amber lighting works wonders for the skin, giving it a warm, soft, creamy look and neutralizing any slight imperfections. Bright white lights have this blue haze, and that's what highlights our skin's flaws, like varicose veins, blemishes, and tired, baggy eyes. Nobody's perfect, but the right lighting can help us feel closer to it!"
>
> —Candida Royalle, pioneer, erotic filmmaker, and author

## GO WITH THE THREAD

If you're doing it on your bed—and by no means should that be the only place you do it—don't neglect your sheets. Seriously, before I became a sheet snob, I couldn't have cared less about cotton, sateen, or silk. Now I buy only three-hundred-thread-count sheets, and I never buy sheets that feel stiff. My three-hundred-plus-thread-count sheets make me feel special, and nicer sheets hug your body in ways that starched cotton can't. Self-pleasure is all about pampering—even in those quickie sessions—and little things, like sheets, can make a big difference.

## MAKE SOME NOISE

Music helps break you out of the quiet zone and put you in a place of auditory freedom. If you use a vibrator while you play, you can quell any anxieties and alleviate fear that your roommates or family might be listening in and, well, hearing you masturbate. Also, music can help you get into a groove, allowing you to free your mind so the rest will follow. Finding a rhythm can help you enjoy the experience, and getting up and dancing before you even begin can help you loosen up even more. Music also allows you to get more vocal, since you can express yourself better and louder with the help of an audio distraction. So go ahead—get comfortable and moan along. Other auditory accompaniments work well, too. Things like porn or erotic audio stories will help turn you on and relax you as you get into the sounds of sex.

> *"I love moaning when I masturbate, and the louder the better. My own moaning turns me on. Is that narcissism?"*
>
> —Sam, age twenty-eight

## SPLISH AND SPLASH

If you're a bath kind of girl, getting into one before you get it on—or getting it on in one—can enhance your solo sexual satisfaction. Add candles, lining them up along the tub, for extra ooh-la-la. A sudsy soak can put your mind in a sensual space, and your skin will feel and smell squeaky clean. And clean skin is fresh skin, which helps when you want to smother your body with self-love. A nice long session of cleansing yourself of your regular thoughts and letting yourself get away from your regular routine is a bubblelicious way to let your stress go down the drain and to comfortably enjoy your present state of being.

## RUB YOURSELF DOWN

While it's not easy to give yourself a two-handed back massage, you can easily rub your feet and arms, your thighs, your neck, and your scalp without the help of a hired hand. So get in the mood by relaxing your body through self-massage. A light, scented oil can smell delicious and really add to the tactile titillation of masturbation. Silicone lube is usually not scented, but it too makes for a great massage, and when you schedule a playdate with a partner, it's condom-compatible as well!

## THE OTHER IN-AND-OUT

Okay, obviously you have to breathe in order to masturbate and, more important, in order to live, but actually paying attention to your breathing can heighten your own levels of arousal. In fact, the more you focus on your breathing, the more relaxed you'll get, and the more relaxed you are, the more sensitive to touch you become. So focus on every breath you take, and allow yourself to get into the zone.

## WET IS THE WORD

You'll want to keep lube around, either water-based or silicone, or even that massage oil (if you're not using any toys and you're basically playing with it on your clit), so that you can reduce the amount of friction that occurs when you touch yourself. Or use spit, it is your own natural lubricant, after all.

## DRESS TO IMPRESS

Again, this isn't something you need to do every time, but we spend more time dressing up for other people than we ever do trying to turn ourselves on. Wear your favorite pair of panties and a matching bra, or a see-through top, or even some thigh-high fishnets and heels. This can help you feel beautiful, boost your self-esteem, and get you visually excited and aroused. Added bonus: Perform a striptease for yourself in front of a full-length mirror and slowly take it all off. Not only will it get you in the mood, but it's great practice for additional foreplay in partnersex.

> *"I sometimes masturbate in front of a mirror so I can watch myself while I do it. It can be a full-length mirror, or a small one that I position in between my legs. I like watching myself get turned on; it's definitely great visual fodder for me!"*
>
> *—Toni, age forty-seven*

## *C* IS FOR COMFORT AND COMING

Wherever you do it, make sure that you're comfortable. If you're on a couch, you might want to prop additional pillows under your back or butt for support. Even if you're on your bed or the floor, pillows are a great help when it comes to happily maneuvering into a variety of positions. Make sure that the thermostat is set at the right temperature for you, or challenge yourself (if you feel like heightening your senses) by making it a tad colder than it should be. Once you start, it's nice to know that everything you're going to use is within arm's reach, so you don't have to get up and get something else out of a drawer, or from under the bed, in order to get off. That means keeping toys, lube, and other sensual items (like feathers, a dildo, or a flogger) nearby, so you can just reach out and grab them.

Getting in the mood does require preparation, but it doesn't necessarily require large amounts of thinking about the perfect scenario. Sometimes you won't want or have time to prepare the perfect night for and with yourself. Quickies are great, too. So is the split-second decision to just do it right then and there, maybe because you've just seen a racy image, shot off a dirty text message, reread a hot email, or need a break. Any excuse you have is a good excuse for release. For some of us, touch, or even the thought of it, is all we need to turn ourselves on and to get our mojo in motion. Once you're in the mood, there are lots of ways you can keep going and going and going.

**GET INTO THE GROOVE**

You're relaxed, settled back, and ready for some one-on-one action. It's always nice when you have the time to take it slow, but again, it's not necessary. Spend as much time as you can appreciating—hell, even worshipping—your body. Start by touching yourself around your neck, your breasts, and your arms. Explore where you have the smoothest patches of skin and the places that leave you feeling more vulnerable. Start with a gentle touch, then move to areas that require more stimulation and apply more pressure. Move down to your belly, pinching, squeezing, rubbing, and loving your tummy. Suck on your fingers and then head south to your mound. Massage the area with circular rubs or press down with your fingers toward your genitals.

Really get to know your vulva. Shake hands with it, cup your hand on top of it, and feel, really feel, the warmth of your beautiful temple. Before you uncover what's beneath, run your fingers up and down the outside of your box. Play with the fleshiness of the outer lips. Notice the amount of hair you do, or don't, have down there. Think about how it feels to tease yourself, to know that very soon you will be heading on inside your family jewels. Imagine how you want to touch and pleasure yourself. Turn yourself on with fantasy. It doesn't have to be anything intricate; just knowing that you're giving yourself permission to love your body can be fodder enough.

Once you've mentally prepared yourself, it's time to gently part your lips with a finger or two. Allow your finger to slowly enter the space between your inner lips, and move it around, up and down, side to side, zig and zag, figuring out the lay of the land. Make your way up to your clit, and notice all of her various parts. Run your hand above the hood, and feel the rubbery cord that is your shaft. Expose your clit even if just for a second, so you understand its sensitivity. Move side to side over the head, gently at first, and then with a little added determination. Play with your clit for a while, then head down to the vagina and lightly tease your opening, and then tease the bit underneath the opening, the place we call the fourchette. Notice how moist you are, and if you're not all that wet, you can always suck on a finger or two for extra lubrication.

How far in do you want to go? Will it be far back, or is a gentle tease with the tip of a finger enough of a feel-good experience? Make a note of where the sensations are the greatest. Does simply suggesting that you may go in invigorate you? Think about how warm you are inside, and explore how the ridgy parts of your vagina feel. Slide a finger or two inside your pussy, and allow yourself to enjoy the feeling of your natural lubrication. Then bring that wetness back up to your clit. Play with different techniques and allow yourself to focus on what's happening in the moment. Concentrate on the shape and size of your clitoris as it gets more and more aroused. Can you feel your genitals congesting with blood?

At this point you should do whatever makes you feel good. You can tug on your lips or touch your breasts. As you get more aroused, you may want to add some vibration or a dildo or butt plug. You can even add all three and stuff yourself silly. If you decide to add buzz, be aware that you can get off really quickly, and, unless your goal is a quick 'gasm, don't let the vibrator seize total control of your arousal—at least not yet. Let it build you up and bring you to a more ecstatic level, and then turn it off. Get back to your hands. Or skip the vibration altogether. Play with your nipples. Build yourself up again without vibration and start doing Kegels, if you haven't been doing them already. When you feel overwhelmed with sensation, find a place that's nice to touch but still won't take you over the edge.

If you do slide a sex toy inside you, make sure you're fully aroused, and make sure the toy is fully lubed. Then gently glide it up inside yourself. You can move it back and forth, or, if you've got a strong PC muscle, hold on to it and lift it up. If it's going up your bum, the more excited you are before you insert it, the better it will feel once it's inside.

As you get closer to orgasm, make sure you're practicing your PC muscle exercises, because they will make a good orgasm even better. Squeeze in, hold, release, repeat. You can also try flicking on your clit at this point; the more aroused you are, the better it feels. Continue with these moves and motions if you want to come. At some point, changing it up may become a downer, but there's nothing wrong with having to rebuild if you've got the time, patience, and willpower.

> *"My favorite masturbation technique is when I use my fingers and a small dildo pressed up against my G-spot. I use the two fingers of my right hand to touch myself, quite rough and fast, especially as the tension builds, but I never go directly onto my clitoris. Then I use my left hand to squeeze my right nipple. I prefer to lie on my back and squeeze my legs at the same time, while I'm also moving my pelvic area up and down to simulate intercourse. My breathing is also important as I get aroused. I close my eyes and try to drift away. It's all in the combination of things together, and the recognition of knowing how I'm about to come, that makes me come."*
>
> —Salka, age thirty-three

 ## THE *M* WORD: MASTURBATION YOUR WAY

There is no right, wrong, one, or best way to masturbate. So forget Simon, Paula, and Randy; they won't be judging you on your techniques, orgasms, or positions. Nobody can feel what you feel the same way you feel it—which is what's so unique about your sexuality. One person's speed pass to sensationville is another person's traffic jam. If you're looking for the road to masturbation, there's only one way to get there, and that's your way.

## THE *HITE REPORT:* MASTURBATION TECHNIQUES

Sex researcher Shere Hite felt that society, culture, and family significantly impacted a woman's view of sex. As a result, she released her *Hite Report* (1976), which focused on how women personally *felt* about sex, rather than showing how statistics, graphs, and charts said they should feel. By providing a more thorough understanding of female sexuality through concentrating on actual experiences, Hite believed women would have a more complete understanding of their own sexual identities. Over the course of four years, a total of 3,019 women contributed to Hite's research, answering more than sixty questions apiece.

Hite asked women about masturbation, including specifics about enjoyment, importance, and technique. Some women, she found, enjoyed it physically but not psychologically; others couldn't enjoy it at all; still others absolutely adored it. Certain women felt masturbation was important as a substitute for partnered sex, while others thought it helped improve their partnered sex. For some, it was a critical tool for learning, independence, and pleasure. Hite also noted that there were six variations of female masturbation, and that 47 percent of women masturbated their clits only. Describing practices ranging from simple manual stimulation of the clitoris to the use of penetration, thrusting, squeezing, rubbing, and vibrating (there was no mention of "rectal stimulation," as she later referred to it), Hite provided a detailed account of how women loved to love themselves.[1]

### CLIT CONTROL

Almost all women masturbate with some form of clitoral stimulation, even the ones who orgasm from penetration. Therefore, let's think of your body as a spaceship and your clit as the most sensitive button on the control panel. You need to know how your clit operates in order to maneuver this craft into orbit. Remember to treat her kindly and check in on her often.

> "My favorite position (probably because I learned to masturbate while reading) is on my stomach with a hand beneath me, and sometimes still with a romance novel in front of me. Through different stages of my life I have experimented with clitoral, vaginal, vaginal and clitoral, and vaginal and anal stimulation. These past couple of years have been all about the clit. It's just easy and less messy."
>
> —Alissa, age twenty-five

Don't make a beeline for the unprotected head of the clit when you masturbate. To test-drive your clit, use whichever hand's most comfortable, and focus the tips of two fingers on the shaft and clitoral hoodie. If you go directly for the head of your clit, you might notice that it's more uncomfortable than it is pleasurable. That's because you're so damn sensitive there—eight-thousand-nerve-endings sensitive! Instead, touch a little to the right or left of the head, and notice if one side is more receptive than the other. Circular motions, or side-to-side ones, generally work well when you're pressing your buttons because they won't expose the clit every time you rub. This'll allow your clit to come out of her shell in her own time. Bonus: To play more easily with your clitty, use your other hand to hold open your lips for better access.

> "I only reach orgasm from clitoral stimulation. It's either sitting down in a chair, sitting on a couch, or lying down in my bed. I usually start by rubbing around in a circle to get myself stimulated, and then I start rubbing up and down on my clitoris when I'm on the verge of having an orgasm."
>
> —Shelly, age thirty-one

**BEGINNER BASICS**

Varying speed, intensity, and types of touch are all good ways to get to know what you really like. Playing with toys and without them will let you know just which tools to use, and experimenting with the mood and positions will help enhance your experience. But if you're just looking for technique, here are some basics.

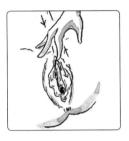 Try using the tips of your fingers or the palm of your hand. Add a little lube or spit to the desired touch utensil and move from side to side, and then up and down (once you're more aroused), and then both, over the head, hood, and shaft of your clit. Wetness, whether generated from down below, from your mouth, or from manufactured lubrication, is going to make this an even smoother ride.

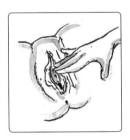 Go the distance. Use your two, three, or four fingers and stroke in between your inner lips, moving up and down like you would with a paintbrush, all the way from the fourchette to the front commissure. Of course, you can stop and start at any other two points, but cover some ground with this one. Don't focus only on your clit.

Take a finger or two and rub circles around your clitoris, making sure to hit a little to the left and a little to the right of the head. Check in with the frenulum and the front commissure from time to time, too. You can do it up big or little, depending on the size of the circles you like. And you can try oodles and oodles of circles, making a chain all the way down to your fourchette and back up to your clit.

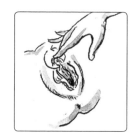

You can basically take any letter or number and try it on for size. Make an S or a V, or spell out the words *masturbation* and *orgasm* and see how that feels. The number eight is a personal favorite because the motion of your fingers teases the vagina and lips, as well as the clit. Visualize the two circles like a forward and backwards S, and notice how there's one spot that gets double love.

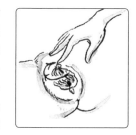

Try this one once you're already aroused and even on the verge of coming. Tap the tips of your fingers on your clitoris, head on, and spank yourself silly, but not too silly; in fact, light love taps might feel incredible at this stage of the game. It may seem a tad bit porny, and it is, but it also feels really good at just the right moment. Optional: Spread your lips back and lift the hood while you do this.

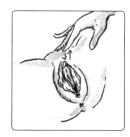

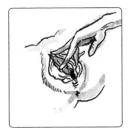

Spread the lips apart with two fingers, and use a third finger to tickle your clitoral landscape. You can lightly flick the area, make small circles, or do whatever you like—it is your clit, after all. Optional: Occasionally make your way down to your vagina, and stick your finger inside. Not only will it feel good, it will also provide additional moisture externally.

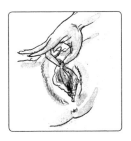

First, try delicately squeezing your clit in between your thumb and index finger. Squeeze, release, squeeze, release. You can also try tugging on your clitoral hood or your vaginal lips. You can—and should—squeeze your PC muscle while you masturbate. This will lead to deeper orgasms, and it provides an added sensation to the base of your genitals.

 **FACT** Masturbation is the way most females (and males) have their first orgasm.[2]

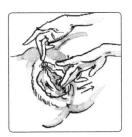

Add penetration. For more stimulation, try gingerly sticking a finger from your other hand into the entrance of your vagina. You can penetrate more deeply with the finger in your pussy, if you like, or just make a circular motion right outside the entryway.

**TIP** No matter how you rub, it doesn't hurt to keep your fingernails clean and trim. This way, the only thing you'll give yourself is pleasure.

 ## BONUS POINTS

When it comes to different strokes for different folks, it's not only about using your hands. How you position yourself can be just as important as what you decide to do in that position. Some women lie on their backs, some women lie on their stomachs, others lie on their sides (or curled up in a ball), and others sit up in a chair. Some women lie with their legs wider apart, some with their legs bent at the knees, others with their thighs pressed together, and others with their legs flat on the bed, toes pointing out. A lot of women keep their legs together because it can increase the sensation of their orgasms. Any way you do it is the right way for you, so choose the position that feels good and get to it.

 ## ON OUR BACKS

Next time you're lying on your back petting the kitty, try out some of the following leg variations for this popular position.

### THE WRAPAROUND
Instead of just bending your knees and keeping your feet flat on the bed, lift your feet and wrap your arms under your knees. In this position you can hold your thighs close to your chest, and give yourself a hug/stretch while you masturbate.

### THE BIG SQUEEZE

Lie flat on your back, with your legs pressed tightly together. Then tickle the ivories while you squeeze and release your thighs (but make sure they keep on touching). Add extra stimulation by practicing your Kegel exercises.

### HEAD TO TOE

Lying on your back, lift your legs so that they're at a ninety-degree angle with your torso (think the letter L). Keep your legs as straight as is comfortable—like when you do lower-abs exercises—and work your magic. Try spreading your legs apart, and then bring your thighs together. You can also lean against a wall for extra support. This is the kind of position where you can observe your reactions from head to toe!

 **ALT-RB8TION**

Since the key to changing up your masturbation routine is imagination, here's a list of techniques to try and things to add to get you out of the bed or off your back. Some of these positions may test your strength, agility, and comfort level.

### FLICK AND FLY

No matter how you stroke your clit or the rest of your vulva, try sitting up and stroking it with your feet in what yogis call the "butterfly." That means with the soles of your feet pressed together and your knees pointing outward, so that each leg looks as if it's in a V shape. Continue pressing the soles of both feet together and playing with your PC muscle at the same time for added enhancement.

## NEED YOUR KNEES

Place pillows underneath both your knees, and masturbate from this kneeling position or vary it up and sit back on your calves. This position isn't comfortable for all women, but it's great for a change-up.

## A TOUCH OF TUMMY

Try masturbating on your stomach with your legs together and/or slightly apart. Without hands, lie on your tummy and rub yourself against an object—even a blanket or pillow can work. Or place one or both of your hands under your body to help you get off.

## RUBBED RIGHT

You don't have to be naked for this one. Try rubbing your vulva against the arm of your sofa, or another soft object. Wear tight undies under your pants and sit down in a chair and rock your hips back and forth. Or head to the gym and work out on your favorite abs machine, or do pull-ups (some women can get off this way). Get daring—find a quiet playground and play on the monkey bars. You don't want to get caught, but trying to get off in a discreet yet public way can be totally hot.

 Rubdown: Rub against a pillow, a towel, your couch, or the armrest in your car and see how that feels up against your clit. Try sitting on the washing machine or enjoying the car's hum as you're driving on the freeway. Try a hands-free rub as you walk in a tight pair of jeans, or put your cell phone down your pants and call yourself often.

## STRENGTHENING AND TONING

Yeah, masturbation can be a workout. But if you want to burn even more calories, try positions that challenge your body. Sit up tall on a bed or couch while your lower body dangles below. Without letting your toes touch the floor, get yourself off. You'll need to use extra strength to keep yourself upright, and this can help tone and strengthen both your leg and stomach muscles. You can also press your feet up against a wall and push up against it to remove your bottom half from the floor. It's a good idea to put a pillow or blanket under your back, both for comfort and to help you avoid sliding (if you have a wooden or slippery floor). Lift and lower your buttocks as you masturbate for additional exercise.

### ROCK OUT

Rock your hips back and forth, or up and down, as you masturbate. It gets the blood flowing and the body going when you move around while you jill off. Even if you're lying on your back, you can still act like you're having partnersex with yourself by thrusting your hips forward as if you're fucking the air.

> "My favorite way to masturbate is to stick an ice cube in my vagina while I play with my clit. I squeeze my pussy muscles as the ice melts inside of me. I love the initial chill of the ice cube, as well as the feeling of the water flowing out of me. My best advice (if you do try this) is to put a towel under you. Otherwise—and depending on where you do it—you may have to sleep in the wet spot."
>
> —Jana, age thirty-seven

### RUB-A-DUB-DUB

The bath, shower, and jacuzzi have helped bring many women to orgasm. Next time you're in the bathtub, place yourself directly under the running water and let it massage your vulva, allowing the rush of warm wetness to hit your clit. If you have a removable showerhead, you can also take the shower nozzle and spray it right on your most sensitive bits. And the bath is a great place to experiment with masturbation and temperature. Start out with a warm stream of water on your clit, and then turn the tap to cold or make it even warmer, and experience the different effects that temperature has on your body. You can also move your body farther from or closer to the faucet, depending on your threshold for pleasure. If you have a pool or hot tub, don't forget the jets. Place yourself in front of one of them and spread your legs wide. Tease yourself. Start farther back and slowly move closer to the actual jet. Notice how the intensity of the stimulation changes depending on your position and your location. Once you try it you'll understand why masturbating in water is one of the most popular ways to come.

### ADD AN EXTRA TOUCH

Rub yourself off with a piece of silk over your clit, or wear a latex glove next time you get off. Let a feather brush against your vulva, or try getting off by playing with yourself over your cotton panties. Get a cheap string of plastic pearls and cut it so that it's one long strand. Then rub the pearls back and forth between your legs, over your clit and vulva.

> *"I'm pretty sure the first time I felt that rush that caused my clitoris to throb was in the bathtub. I figured out how to position my clitoris directly under the running water from the faucet, and I would hold it there until I could feel the orgasm coming. I remember that the water caused me to rock back and forth, and I loved the sensation of relaxing and letting go. I can't remember how old I was, maybe eight or nine, but I will always remember the orgasm."*
>
> *—Allison, age twenty-four*

## MASTURBATION AND PIERCINGS

Can genital piercings enhance masturbation? Yes! Sexual pleasure is, after all, the point of getting them. Lots of women say that piercings increase sensation, which often leads to more intense orgasms.

The easiest, least painful, and most sensational genital piercing for women is the vertical clitoral hood piercing. This piercing runs parallel to the clitoral shaft, so that the bottom part of the piercing hits the clit. Another popular piercing is the horizontal clitoral hood piercing, which passes through the clitoral hood horizontally above the clit. It doesn't provide much stimulation for the clit, but for piercing fans it sure looks pretty. A triangle piercing requires that the jewelry be inserted below the hood and behind the clit, and it stimulates both the back and the front of the clit.

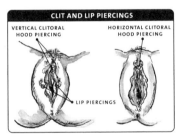

**CLIT AND LIP PIERCINGS**

VERTICAL CLITORAL HOOD PIERCING

HORIZONTAL CLITORAL HOOD PIERCING

LIP PIERCINGS

If someone has a true clit piercing, that means she has a piercing running through her clitoris. Other options for piercing include the inner or outer lips and the fourchette.

Not all women are built for genital piercings, and just because you have a clit doesn't mean it's the right size or shape to get a metal rod or hoop pushed through it. So don't get your heart set on a particular type of piercing before you do your research. You'll want to check with a good, hygienic piercing professional. (Do not make any sudden decisions with a sleazy piercer guy.) You won't be able to masturbate, or have any other form of sex, until your new buddy is completely at home in your body, which can mean between four and eight weeks.

## PLAYING WITH TOYS

Giving yourself a helping hand during masturbation is more than okay. It can change up the way you have sex with yourself big time—whether it's a five-minute fix or an hour of pleasure. Yippee!

If you don't get totally wet from the sheer thought of touching yourself, or from stimulating yourself with your hands for a while, you'll definitely want to grab some lube. Make sure you're comfortable, and start by warming yourself up with your hands. That means fondling around beyond the clit—on the lips, the breasts, the nape of your neck, any place you find erotic. You can always go straight for the vibrator, but it's just not as much fun as turning yourself on before you take out the toys.

If you're going to use a dildo, start out slow. Once you're lubed up and ready, insert a finger into your pussy as a way to introduce your vagina to outside forces. After you've noticed the sensations you can bring to yourself by working on your own body, you can replace the finger with a dildo. But first, fuck yourself with a finger, moving in and out, round and round, and in any other formation that works for you. Go all the way in, and all the way back out. Stay focused on the entrance to the vagina, press down on the bottom wall of the vagina, and press up on the top wall near your G-spot.

If you're playing with a dildo, you can place it inside yourself and press your PC muscle around it to stimulate your entire pelvic floor. Try a weighted dildo, like the Energie or Betty's Barbell, which work as Kegel exercisers and also make great playthings.

If you're using a vibrator check out how it feels on and off your clit. Use it on the outside of your lips and on your perineum. Have a separate vibe ready for your bum (if you like backdoor fun!). If it's long, test out the vibration on the inside of your body. See where you feel it the most. If it's curved, hook it around to your G-spot (even though straight vibes can hit the spot too), or just play with the sensations internally. (Refer back to "How to Hit the G-spot" on page 23.) You can even put on vibrating or non-vibrating nipple clamps for sensation above the belt, then go back to working on your below-the-belt antics.

You can play with household items, too, like an electric toothbrush (you may want to cover the bristles with plastic wrap first) or a hairbrush (please be gentle with this one, and only use one that's dedicated to masturbation and not to brushing your hair as well). Make sure that whatever you use is clean and can be cleaned after each use.

If you're ready for butt stimulation, take a finger vibe (lots of them come with multiple sleeves, so you can have one that fits over its head for vaginal play and one for anal play) and rub it around your rectum. When you're totally turned on, move a lubed (non-vibrating) finger up your butt and relax into it. Then move on to bigger things, like a plug—silicone is nice and easy to clean—and slide it up in there. Again, lube is required. Leave the plug in place and then go back to stimulating your clit. Penetrate yourself with a dildo and see how that feels while you have something else up your bum. You can always increase the size of your butt toy if you feel like it, but start slow and build up toward that. Keeping something up your bum while you masturbate your front bits does provide extra stimulation, sensation, and pleasure if ass play is something you like. So experiment with toys to see what you like and don't like. And if you don't want to use toys to get off, or in conjunction with getting off in other ways, don't worry. Like I said, while it can open the door to whole new experiences, it's not for everyone.

 ## DOUBLE YOUR PLEASURE: DOING IT TOGETHER

Okay, fine; up till now I've been touting the benefits of sex for one because solo sexual gratification is the most important type of sex you can have with yourself. Getting to know your body is an integral part of your existence on a sexual, physical, and psychological level. Finding out what makes you go *tick tick boom* is more important than having anybody else manufacture your orgasmic explosions. First and foremost, it's best to know your own body and to not let anybody else take responsibility for your pleasure. But that's not to say that you won't learn a lot from having sex with others (or at least another), or that you shouldn't have partnersex, or a partner—and that doesn't mean your partner can't get you off, because it's ideal that he or she would. It just means that you need to assume responsibility for your own body, including your own sensuality and sexuality. And in teaching yourself about touch, you can also teach your partner about how you like to be touched (and they don't have to lay a hand on you to learn). Yep, that's right—it's called mutual masturbation, and it's not only hot, exciting, and voyeuristic, it's also a fantastic partnersex teaching tool.

> "I think it's a real turn-on to watch my partner masturbate. It reflects the level of comfort the relationship has reached and the comfort he has with his own body. You get a very intimate peek at exactly what he does, his movements, his speed, the ways he gets off, and you know he's turned on by you watching. It's kind of flattering, actually."
>
> —Lindsay, age twenty-two

Unfortunately, lots of girls aren't into their partners' wanking off when they're not around, just like lots of guys and girls don't want their women to use vibration or jill off manually when they aren't doing the job themselves. But honestly, it's time we all grow up and get over these insecurities and hangups, and accept and honor the fact that we are not the only people our partners seek pleasure from, and vice versa. Being in a relationship doesn't mean you give up your individuality—in your sex life or any other endeavor. Instead, embrace the fact that your partner likes to touch him- or herself, and still maintains control of his or her body. Use this knowledge to empower yourself and build upon your arsenal of tricks and techniques that will enhance your lover's moans and motions and ensure their rock-solid orgasms. Think of mutual masturbation as a front-row ticket to your favorite concert—it's a backstage pass, a VIP invitation, and an exclusive offer. And that's what makes it so damn good.

Even if you're not convinced, and especially if you are, give it a go at least once and see how you feel and what you learn—if and when you have a partner to practice with. If you have hangups about doing it, or watching your partner do it, make it a special night. Prepare by setting the mood in a romantic, candlelit sort of way. You might want to do a joint activity before or after, or promise each other that after you each have your first self-made orgasm, you'll make a go at it together. Think about and discuss whatever you need to in order to assure yourself that this doesn't make you any less important, relevant, or necessary in your partner's sex life. And really understand that it doesn't, and then let it all go, and be there, present, with your partner, ready to do it together, yet alone.

## ON YOUR MARK, GET SET, MASTURBATE

Before you begin, make sure there's lube around, because masturbation goes smoother if you have it on hand. You might want to begin with a little striptease for yourself and each other. If you've ever been to a strip club or a burlesque show, then you'll know that much, if not all, of the sexual buildup comes in the form of seductive removal of clothing—or sometimes, in the case of certain strip clubs, the less seductive, rip 'em-right-off-and-dance-around-topless approach. Bringing your partner to your special place will feel less isolating if you make sure to include him or her in your foreplay. So seductively remove a few layers of clothes for each other, and make sure to establish eye contact along the way, and throughout the entire experience. That doesn't mean you'll always look each other in the eyes, but it does mean you want to make sure you connect with your partner on a visual level. Make sure that your partner's aware of being watched, and even if, as you climb to the point of ecstasy, you have to shut your eyes and throw your head back, make a mental note to open them every so often and have a good look at the person you care about, who's experiencing their own pleasurable ride right next to you.

> "We often do the mutual masturbation thing. I've learned how to get him off better as a result, and I don't mind him masturbating on his own without me, even though I'm not sure if he does—I mean, I've asked him and he says he doesn't. Still, I don't hide the fact that I masturbate from him, and I generally get off by masturbating in front of him after he fucks me. It's our little sex habit."
>
> —Elizabeth, age thirty-seven

Try some different positions. You can sit across the room from each other for a truly hands-off (each other), hands-on (yourselves) experience, or you can sit next to each other and touch each other while you do it. That means things like caressing your partner's legs or arms, or maybe playing with their hair, as you get off. One person can also straddle the other, allow-

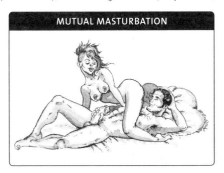

**MUTUAL MASTURBATION**

ing a few up-close-and-personal moments of visual pleasure. Alternately, you can hang out in a version of visual 69. That means you'll be giving each other pleasure without touching one another. The partner on top should be in doggie style with his or her butt dangling over the chest or head of the partner on the bottom. The person on bottom is lying on their back. In this position you get to play with yourself while watching your partner do the same. It's like two for the price of one!

**ADDED EXCITEMENT**

**Play with toys.** If you're into vibration or shoving something else up your twat, or bum, as you climb to the climax, don't shy away from going there now. It will turn your partner on to know where they can go when getting you off as well. And if you're dating a dude, don't assume that he doesn't want to play with toys. A guy who hasn't tried vibration on his balls, on his shaft, on his perineum, and around his asshole doesn't know what he's been missing out on. Give him a vibe to play with—either brand-new, or one that you don't both use for penetration. You can even put a condom on the toy so that sharing isn't a problem. And if he's into ass play, give him something that will stimulate his prostate, like an Aneros prostate stimulator, which will allow him to keep a toy up his butt while he keeps his hands on his dick.

**Moan if you want to.** While noise or words can sometimes sound fake and phony, the more you say them and the more you mean them, the less pornorrific they become. Even if you just moan a little, you're providing your own audio enticement, and that will be a turn-on for both you and your partner. If you can't get yourself to go there, perhaps a CD of dirty stories, like the ones from Sounds Erotic, will provide additional entertainment for the two of you. Or practice in front of a mirror before your mutual masturbation playdate. Saying things over and over again will make it feel more natural.

**Move around a little, or a lot.** Even if when you're alone you lie like a log when you come, moving your hips and setting your body in motion will add extra visual stimulation. Not to mention that masturbation maven Betty Dodson thinks that pelvic movement is integral to great masturbation. So give it a try, both for your own pleasure and for your partner's visual delight.

## CROSSING THE FINISH LINE

Announce when you're coming. A lot of times, once you really get into your groove, you lose a sense of space and time and forget where you are or why you're there. The orgasm you're about to give yourself, and the orgasm your partner is about to have, are the pinnacle moments in your mutual masturbation endeavor. By announcing your arrival before it happens, you're allowing your partner the ultimate in VIP moments, and therefore you want to make sure they don't miss a beat. Give them at least ten seconds to get back to this planet (they may be off on their own journey at this point) and let them know that you want them to watch you finish yourself off. Bonus points: Try to look them in the eyes when you come.

If you finish first, allow your partner the time they need to have their first orgasm without your showing any signs of irritation or discomfort. Find ways to encourage them in their venture. If you're not already sitting close to your partner, get closer and whisper words of encouragement— things like "You're so hot" or "I love watching you touch yourself"—to help maintain the momentum and assuage any anxiety they may be feeling now that the spotlight's completely on them. Rub their head, tweak their nipples, and kiss their neck in an effort to cheer for the team. You can even start playing with yourself again if you so please.

Mutual masturbation is the best way to get to know what your partner likes, while showing your partner what you like too. It's not a threatening act and it's not wrong. After it's done you'll most likely feel closer to your partner than you did before.

Mutual masturbation is all about you, even when it's about your finding ways to show your partner how you please yourself. It's not about what feels good to someone else, and it's not about guilt or shame. Masturbation is healthy. It's natural. It's instinctual. So go with the flow and get moving your own way, in your own time, with your own style!

 **QUICKIES: TIPS FOR TOUCHING**

- Start slowly, allowing yourself to really feel who you are and what you're doing.

- Light candles to help set the mood.

- If you rub over the clitoral hood from side to side and not up and down, you're exposing less of the (sometimes way too sensitive) clit in the early stages of arousal.

- Make circles around your clitoris and come in contact with more surface area in the region that surrounds it.

- Push down on the front commissure and feel the clitoral shaft underneath it.

- Practice your Kegel exercises to improve your orgasmic potential.

- Try masturbating while you're fully dressed by rubbing your cunt up against a piece of furniture or by sitting on your washing machine.

- Masturbate in front of a mirror and notice how your genitals change as you get more aroused, and watch how you turn yourself on.

- Make noise and talk dirty to yourself. Tell yourself how beautiful you are, how hot your body is, how good you feel. Build up your sexual self-esteem so that you can feel good during partnersex as well!

- Let your imagination run wild and go with your fantasies, politically correct or not.

- Tease yourself. Go to the point where you could come, and then stop and bring yourself back down again. Then turn up the volume. Try doing this a few times before you let yourself go, and see if your orgasms intensify.

- The more you masturbate, the more in touch you'll be with your body and the more you'll enjoy other sex as well.

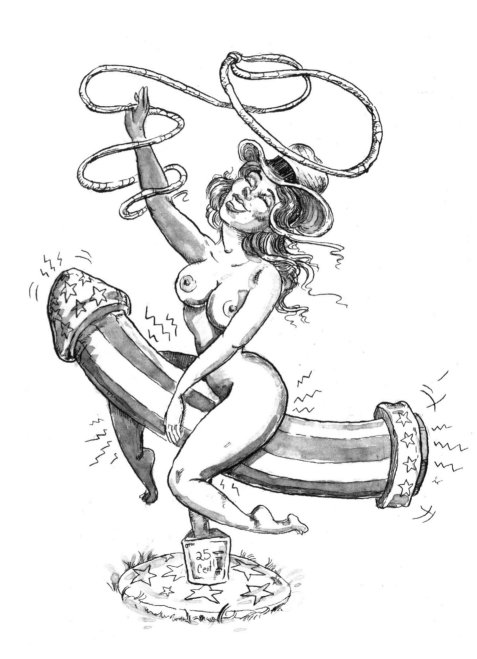

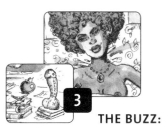

### THE BUZZ:
### *Everything You Ever Wanted to Know About Vibrators*

ALMOST EVERY WOMAN, whether she's a seasoned pro or a curious newbie, has heard the word *vibrator*. This buzzing or oscillating sex toy is an essential and integral part of a woman's individual sexploration, and without the vibrato of vibration many women would never have been able to climb to their personal peaks. I am a member of the tribe that adores their vibes, and I realize that my life would not be the same without the magic of manufactured sensation. My first orgasm, at the age of twenty-one, came after years of having partnered sex and continuously wondering whether I had actually come. Yep, only after having my first battery-powered orgasm did I realize that I was finally a member of Club "O." To this day I owe a lot of my sexual exploration, and many, many orgasms, to vibrators (especially the Pocket Rocket and the Eroscillator).

If you're not sure what the difference is between a vibrator and a dildo, here's the lowdown. A vibrator vibrates; a dildo does not—or at least it's not required to. Nowadays there are dildos that come with vibrating attachments, but the general rule of thumb is that when something needs batteries, or plugs into a wall, it's generally called a vibrator. Also, a vibrator is not something that has to be inserted inside your pussy or your ass in order to get you off. It can be small and stylish, and used primarily on your clit, or even your vaginal lips. A dildo is an insertable object that goes in one of two holes, and it's designed for pushing your buttons during penetration.

Vibrators are like the high school football team or the cheerleading squad of sex toys. They are the most popular toys on the market, and they get the most attention because they can boost morale, provide excitement, and perk us up when we're feeling down. For a lot of women, vibrators are an indispensable piece of the orgasmic puzzle, and even though vibration doesn't do it for all women, plenty are curious enough to at least see what the buzz is about. According to a 2004 survey by Durex, 46 percent of women own a vibrator.[1]

*Sex and the City* officially outed the vibe, and now everybody who's anybody knows about vibration. By making the vibrator that much more socially acceptable, the show succeeded in allowing even the shiest of women to be comfortable with needing or wanting vibration to get themselves turned on. As this appreciation for vibration continues to grow, so does the market that manufactures such products. In the past few years we have seen the emergence of companies that offer classier, higher-end sex toys, ones that allow personal indulgence, pampering, and pleasure. These vibes all come at a price, but they're being researched and designed to work harder to please you.

Some companies spend years manufacturing their toys, working closely with sex therapists to produce the best designs possible. Some of these toys give you more options than your cable TV, while others are built with motors in both ends so that you can get off from any angle. One vibe, the Je Joue, comes with its own PleasureWare software and feels more human than machine. Some boast the tiniest of details. Whether the toy is etched with art or made from aircraft-quality metals, more and more mechanical engineers, sex researchers, and geeks are finding ways to make pleasure better. And even adult novelty companies, the kind of factories that output hundreds of toys a year, including penis pumps and blow-up dolls (adult novelty companies are generally considered the makers of lesser-quality products), keep producing cooler-looking, better-acting, and higher-functioning vibes in order to keep up with the demand.

 ## A SHORT HERSTORY OF VIBRATION

The original vibrators weren't as suggestive as our modern-day phallus-shaped or realistic-looking ones. In fact, most of them were big and bulky, and their bits and pieces resembled some sort of project that a mad scientist could design in their lab, and not something that you'd want to put anywhere near your clit. Still, they worked—and because they never got tired, and consistently provided good vibrations, women loved them.

Vibrators were first used by doctors to treat women for hysteria, a condition that was once considered a disease but whose diagnosis is now outdated and unused. For centuries, starting in Egypt in 2000 BC and in the Western world with Hippocrates in the fifth century BC,[2] hysteria was the most common medical diagnosis for anything off kilter in women. And even though it's not used anymore, if it weren't for hysteria, it's likely that men wouldn't have worked so hard to make vibrating treatment devices— and we might never have known the wonders of vibration. And then who knows where we'd be today?

The first patent for a steam-powered vibrator was granted to an American doctor named George Taylor in 1869. It was large, bulky, and expensive and used only by medical doctors to "cure" their patients. In 1880, the Weiss company manufactured the first battery-operated vibrating apparatus, and within fifteen years of the introduction of this lighter and less costly model, there were more than a dozen other manufactured makes and models of vibration.[3]

By the turn of the twentieth century, vibrators were fast becoming more affordable and available. Physicians' offices were stocked with foot-powered models, or vibes like the larger, more expensive Chattanooga which was fueled by a coal-powered furnace and required two men to operate it. The Hitachi Magic Wand of its day, it was a whopping $200—not a cheap device for the early 1900s.[4]

Vibrators became so popular that they were the fifth appliance to be electrified, following the sewing machine, the fan, the teakettle, and the toaster.[5] By 1900, most of the smaller vibrators were either battery-operated or plug-in. The most popular vibe of that time was the White Cross Electric Vibrator, manufactured by the Lindstrom Smith Company of Chicago. From 1902 through the 1930s, these vibes were marketed as personal massagers that women could use in the privacy of their own home (meaning no more doctor's visits in order to get off).

When vibes first went mainstream, they were marketed as "home appliances" in paid advertisements in popular women's magazines like *Woman's Home Companion, McClure's, Needlecraft,* and *Popular Mechanics.* Even the Sears, Roebuck and Company electrical goods catalog sold its own vibrator, one that multitasked—meaning it had attachments for vibration as well as other useful "womanly" tasks like mixing, beating, and churning.[6] They were supposed to help cure disease, bring blood to the skin's surface, and improve overall health.[7] The vibrator was having its first fifteen minutes of fame, and it was so cool and popular that women all over the country were shopping for vibes through ads in their favorite women's magazines. That is, until all those ads disappeared.

What happened to the vibe? In the late 1920s, early stag films like *Widow's Delight* started showing women using vibrators in all their special places, and vibrators became a star attraction in mainstream porn.[8] Thus, upon the vibrator's theatrical debut, vibrator ads disappeared from "respectable" journals and the vibrator went underground until the late 1950s. Once the vibe made its glorious comeback, there was no beating around the bush and there was no denying that the bush was, in fact, the primary thing women wanted their vibrators for.

**THE IMPORTANCE OF BEING VIBRATIONAL**

The vibrator is the most popular sex toy on the market today, and it's not about to lose its buzz anytime soon. Most women require some form of direct clitoral stimulation to actually get off, and vibration makes it fun and easy to reach that goal. That doesn't necessarily mean you'll want to tackle the clit head-on (you might want to start a little to the right or a little to the left), but it does mean that penetration is not the be-all, end-all when it comes to sex.

> *"I use a vibe every so often. I use it because it's consistent in its abilities. Period. There is no getting tired, and when I'm doing it, I can control the pressure better. Plus, I hate it when my hands get tired."*
>
> —*Lara, age thirty-two*

Some women have a really hard time getting off, or need a really long time before they reach climax. And while you can use your hand or another blunt object, it's easy to get tired and give up the fight. For women who don't come from penetration alone (and that would be 70 percent of us), or for others who have wrist problems, using a vibrator helps make the task at hand that much easier. And if you've never had an orgasm, the right vibrator can absolutely help you achieve your goal.

> *"For a lot of women, a vibrator is an essential part of their sex life. For many women a vibrator is a guaranteed orgasm."*
>
> —*Rachel Venning, cofounder, Babeland*

## SHAPES AND SIZES AND COLORS, OH MY!

Like women, vibrators come in all variations when it comes to how they look, feel, and function. The right vibe for you may not do anything for your best friend—even if she looks and acts just like you. There's no way to look at a vibe, or any sex toy for that matter, and immediately know that it will, or won't, do the trick. Unfortunately, you don't really know until you try, and even once you try, you might not be certain that this is *the one*. But you don't need *the one* to have a good time. Most of the time you'll simply want a vibe that will help you achieve whatever your goal is without overstimulating or understimulating certain body parts.

### THE LONG AND THE SHORT OF IT

Length doesn't generally matter when it comes to vibration; it's way more about the power and the position. A lot of women who like vibration use vibes directly on their clits, so even if you're using something else—a dildo or whatever you're into—inside you, it's your clit that really enjoys the vibrational attention. When choosing your vibrator, go with something that gives you a little bit of power, or the ability to adjust the strength, rather than going for something just because it looks good. And while even the smallest sensation is way too much for some women, don't limit yourself to one setting, at least not at first. A vibe that's on the long side can double as a dildo, which means two bangs for your buck, even if not every woman wants to get banged by her vibe. The long and the short of it is this: You want something that feels good without numbing your clit, and something you'll enjoy using for as long as it lasts.

When considering length, you'll also want to think about curvature. Lots of vibes have a defined upward hook at the tip, and are marketed as G-spot specials. These are shaped like a kinder, softer version of Captain Hook's metal hand. Other vibes look like penises, cell phones, zoo animals, or alien life forms. Sometimes these too curve upward at the end, as if pointing directly toward the sky. While these vibrators are great for helping you hit the spot (either with or without vibration), they're not as much of a selling point as, say, variable speeds, pulsation, or a quiet vibe. However, if you're all about finding the G-spot, it doesn't hurt to have a toy that's specifically for that.

 Courts in Georgia, Mississippi, Alabama, and Texas continue to uphold a ban on the sale of sex toys.

## SETTING THE PACE

A lot of vibes offer variable speeds, and if you're not sure what you like, it's nice to be able to go from soft and slow to hard and fast whenever you feel like it. A vibe with a range of speeds will allow you to tease yourself longer, which can, if desired, result in a nice, lengthy session. You can build yourself up and let yourself down as much as you'd like, and continuously set your own pace as you go at it for the long haul. Or you can keep it on high and get off in a flash. It's your choice. Still, I love the one speed because it allows me to not think about my settings and sensations. One-speed vibes get the job done (as long as you're okay with the speed they're at), even though they limit your ability to tease and please.

> "I've had a variety of vibrators. I use them for clitoral stimulation, and they all have several speeds. I like to start off with a low speed and then end on a high speed."
>
> —Ilene, age twenty-six

## MANNING THE CONTROLS

It's also important to figure out your preferences when it comes to controlling your toy. Some vibes have a simple switch—on or off—while others have slides that allow you to gently upgrade the speed. Some have a rotating dial at the base so you can control them from below, and still others have a separate controller/battery pack that is attached to the vibrating toy by a wiry cord. Some varieties have an unattached battery pack that controls the vibration remotely, from up to twenty or thirty feet away. This last one is awesome for partnered sex too—especially when you're wearing a pair of remote-controlled vibrating panties, or playing with yourself in an environment that necessitates your being hands free, like a restaurant or club. Some people don't care as much about how their vibe is controlled as they do about the style or shape. But some vibes are harder to handle than others, and you want to make sure that in the middle of a good masturbation session, you're the one in control of your plaything.

## POWER SUPPLY

Every year more and more rechargeable vibes find their way onto the market, and they're becoming increasingly popular because they don't require the user to keep batteries in the drawer of her bedside table. Thus, they're not only convenient but cost-effective—and environmentally conscious (with no batteries to throw away, they're more ecofriendly). Plus, you're not confined to masturbating near an electrical outlet like you are with plug-in vibes. Of course, certain plug-ins have really long cords, and you could always use an extension cord to go farther, but cords do tangle. Rechargeable vibes do, however, require that you plan ahead, since you have to make sure the vibe has juice before you give it a go; but other than that, they're easy to use and will last, on average, an hour at a time.

When it comes to battery-operated vibes, some take your standard, bulky C batteries, but most require AA or AAA. Cheapie vibes, more often called adult novelty toys, are generally battery operated, and smaller vibes, like the ones you can wear on your finger, usually take standard watch batteries. Watch batteries never seem to last as long, or feel as powerful, and while it's easy (and cheaper) to buy multiple packs of teeny-tiny batteries online, I'd recommend going with a first vibrator that requires standard AA or AAA batteries, simply because they're so available and offer a wider range of vibration.

**TIP** In order to ensure the life of your vibe, don't leave the batteries in your buddy when you're not at play. This way your toy won't accidentally turn itself on and burn itself out, which can literally spoil your buzz.

Plug-ins are way old-school in style, but for women who like power, these are no joke. Often marketed as back massagers, plug-in vibes generally have two speeds: "wow" and "yowser." Some of them come equipped with vibratodes, a fancy name for attachments that allow the user to choose her own vibration. The most famous plug-in vibe, and one of the most well-known vibes ever, is the Hitachi Magic Wand. Labeled the "Cadillac of vibrators" by its beloved legions of fans, it's the kind of vibe you might want to try with your panties still on because it's just that darn powerful. Oh, and the Magic Wand and most other quality plug-ins come with a one-year limited manufacturer's warranty. How's that for customer satisfaction?

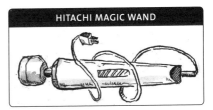

HITACHI MAGIC WAND

> *"I use the Hitachi Magic Wand, but I often feel that the vibrations are too strong, and sometimes my clit feels beat up. It does get me off, but I actually prefer the stimulation of my finger. With my finger it takes longer for me to come, but I come harder and the orgasm is more of an arc than a momentary shudder."*
>
> —Selena Fire, age forty-seven

 ## DUAL DUTIES

Some women think that dual-action vibes (yes, the very same ones made popular by Charlotte on *Sex and the City*), are the be-all, end-all of the vibrational universe. Dual-action vibes bring you pleasure in not one, but two, places. Not only do you get clitoral stimulation with these playthings, but dual-action vibes also penetrate the user while they vibrate, pulsate, twist, and shake (unfortunately, they won't take out the garbage or kiss you or cuddle). Dual-action vibes often consist of two separate parts that are fused together at the same base. They usually have a large shaft for internal penetration and a smaller clitoral stimulator for external stimulation. At the bottom of the base you'll generally find the battery compartment, which can consist of one shared controller—or two switches, buttons, or knobs—for the clitoral stimulator and the vaginal stimulator. Depending on the device, the two parts can be used separately or simultaneously. Oftentimes the clitoral stimulator vibrates while the shaft rotates, and you can generally get at least two inches of penetration before you're actually hitting your clit with the clitoral stimulator. In order to reap the rewards of double stimulation, you have to insert the shaftlike rod into your pussy, which allows the tinier clitoral stimulator to reach your clit. The shaft can look like a penis, or it can resemble a long, straight, or curved sticklike thing-amajig. The clitoral stimulators often resemble animals, and certain parts of each animal—like rabbit ears, a koi tail, or a beaver's tongue—are what specifically work the clitoral region. The most famous of these dual-action vibes is the Rabbit Habit, and while there are more than a few bunnies on the market, the highest quality dual-action toys hail from Japan and a company called Vibratex. Other dual-action vibes are super-curved one piece toys that tend to resemble the letter U. You insert one end of the hooked toy inside you and simply place the other end on your clit. With these U-shaped toys, you may need to rock back and forth to get both ends stimulated. Two popular U-shaped vibes are the Ultime and the Rock-Chick.

## THE VIBRATOR CURSE

An ugly rumor has been making the rounds, one that claims that too much vibration causes a clit to go numb and never ever find its original sensitivity again. And while this is totally scary, it's also absolutely not true. The truth is that your clit will not become desensitized, or incapable of receiving other forms of pleasure, even if you become addicted to vibration. If you get used to coming with a vibrator, it's possible that you won't come as quickly, or even as easily, during partnered sex or masturbation sans vibrator, but this "problem" comes with a simple solution. If you stop using a vibrator, or even if you switch to a less powerful model, you'll soon regain the same level of sensitivity that you originally had in your clit. Of course, not all women are clit-sensitive to begin with, so if you found it difficult to orgasm without a vibrator before, then odds are that will remain true. But if you enjoy other forms of sexual touch (whether with hands, tongues, other toys, or a cock), then limiting the use of your vibrating lover will open the floodgates and allow you to get off, vibration-free, once again.

## WHY PHTHALATE-FREE IS A GOOD THING

The most common material for inexpensive, soft sex toys is jelly rubber. Unfortunately, a majority of these jelly rubber toys contain phthalates (pronounced *thalates*). Phthalates are chemical substances used to make polyvinyl chloride (PVC, which is a type of plastic commonly used for sex toys) soft and flexible. Aside from the fact that phthalates smell awful, studies have shown that they are potentially bad for your health, and can possibly mess with the human reproductive system.[9] So even though these jelly rubber toys might be the best option for your budget, they are not necessarily the best option for your box.

There is good news, though. Some of the larger adult manufacturers, like Topco and Doc Johnson, have said that they will work to eliminate phthalates from production in the future. For now, if you like your jelly rubber toys, then purchase a few extra condoms so that you can safely, and confidently, put the toy inside your vagina (if that is indeed its intended purpose). For clitoral stimulation, it's less of a big deal, but it's still better to be safe than sorry.

Although lots of big toy manufacturers think the hype around phthalates is just that, there are companies jumping off the phthalate-filled-jelly-rubber bandwagon once and for all. Adam and Eve, a large company that specializes in the sale and production of adult movies, sex toys, and lingerie through both online and mail-order catalogs, will stop selling phthalate-filled toys by 2008.[10] Other big toy companies, like Doc Johnson, an adult novelty company that's been selling its own line of sex toys for over thirty years, have introduced a new material they call sil-a-gel, which is still a lower-end sex toy material, but one that's free of the toxic-grade phthalates (though it still contains other phthalates). There are other soft options, too, like silicone and elastomers that do not contain phthalates, but you will pay a higher price for those products. (For a list of other materials on the market, see chapter

4, "Self-Love and Sex Toys.") Unless the packaging on a soft rubber toy states that it's phthalate-free, assume that it's not, and act accordingly.

When in doubt, hard plastic gives great head, and it's truly my favorite way to go. I've tried a lot of different vibrating toys, and when I want it quick and easy, I always go back to my tiny, hard plastic Pocket Rocket or Water Dancer (the waterproof version of the Pocket Rocket), especially when I want to get the job done efficiently and effectively. The Water Dancer and the Pocket Rocket are both small (as in a few inches longer than an average middle finger), one speed (giving you two options, on or off), hard, and nonphallic clitoral stimulators. Of course, I should warn you that most hard plastic vibes get louder over time, so if noise is an issue, hard plastic is not necessarily the solution. However, using any hard plastic vibe under your nice warm blanket (assuming you live in a place where nice warm blankets are needed) will eliminate some noise, as will turning on your stereo or TV. And if noise doesn't bother you, go hard at least once, and check out the sensation.

---

### THE GREAT PHTHALATE DEBATE

Two studies recently conducted about the presence of phthalates in sex toys, one by the Danish Technological Institute (DTI) and one by Greenpeace Netherlands,[11] did not actually prove a link between health issues and phthalate use in humans, even though the Greenpeace U.K. website did seem to overtly imply that there was one. Because safety is important, and even if this all sounds a bit alarmist, I encourage you to go and actually take a whiff of one of these toys (the worse the smell, the more phthalates it contains). Jelly rubber toys have burned women's insides and they do smell toxic. Honestly, if it were up to me, I'd ban jelly rubber toys completely. Still, only you can decide what you want to put in your body, and therefore it's up to you to decide if jelly rubber is right for you.

## A WHOLE LOT OF CHOICES

There are way too many vibes to list here, so instead I've chosen to compile some of the most popular, most interesting, and most unique vibes you can buy. If none of these vibes do it for you, just log on to any of the sex-toy stores listed in chapter 9 and find one that does.

### HARDER, HARDER

The following popular vibes are all hardheaded, and therefore give great buzz. Plus, they're nonporous, they don't smell, and they're easy to clean with soap and warm water.

### •••POCKET ROCKET•••

The Pocket Rocket (Doc Johnson) is probably the most popular tiny, clit-centric vibrator on the market. While it's not as tiny as the Fukuoku 9000, which you'd wear on your finger, it's smaller than the hard, long, and smooth Slimline (Adam and Eve). The Pocket Rocket is one of those lipstick-

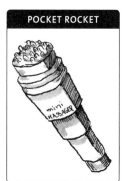

size, four-inch minimassagers that comes with a clear plastic removable tip, fits in your purse or your pocket, has one speed, and makes a bit of noise. It twists on and off and requires one AA battery. The more you use it the louder it gets, but it's a great, easy to handle, easy to use vibe. Its waterproof cousin, the Water Dancer (Vibratex), can be used in the bath or shower. For a different experience, you can add a rabbit sleeve, which looks just like the clitoral stimu-lator on the Vibratex Rabbit Habit. The sleeve's got a hollow bottom and it's made of soft jelly rubber, so it's easy to insert over your Pocket Rocket or Silver Bullet vibe. Then use the ears to tickle your clitty, and you might actually hear her purr.

### •••FUKUOKU 9000•••

The Fukuoku 9000 (Fukuoku) is a hard plastic finger vibe that comes with three silicone sheaths to place on its head. The three attachments have slightly different designs (one has a circle, one has dots, and one has lines), but they all feel the same. Still, if you're sharing your toy with a partner, or using it for stimulation around your bum and your pussy, it's nice to have multiple attachments. While not nearly as powerful as the Pocket Rocket, it doesn't require you to hold on to anything to get your groove on. You just slip it over your finger, and *bam,* you've got a vibrating finger. The actual vibe is hard plastic and lightweight, and the stimulation tips are all silicone. The softer sleeves make the toy feel a little less like hard plastic, but when you wear it you kind of feel like your finger's in a splint. It takes two watch batteries and comes in cool colors; it's also got a number of accessories, including a little black bag to store all the bits. It's not intimidating, and it won't blow the roof off your clit.

### •••EGG VIBRATORS•••

A Silver Bullet (Doc Johnson) is just one of many small vibrating eggs on the market. The egg is literally the shape of a hard-boiled egg, but it's generally a mini version of what a chicken would lay. The color can be silver (hence the name) or white, or it can glow in the dark. Most eggs come with a separate battery compartment (it takes two AA batteries) that's connected to the toy via a long, thin wire. This means that you can place the controller away from your body as the egg stimulates your erogenous zones. Some battery packs come in certain shapes, like a car shape, and others are simple, nothing more than a sliding switch. Eggs also come in both hard and soft varieties. The Silver Bullet is a hard egg vibe, but there are a number of bullets that are softer and smaller and more closely resemble a bloated Tic Tac than an actual egg. These are generally watch battery–operated and don't always have a separate battery pack. Those without the controller usually click on and off via a soft black button on one end. Eggs that require a cord can be less reliable than those without, especially since you're shit out of luck if the cord breaks.

> "My preferred method of masturbation is clitoral stimulation with the bullet vibrator. I keep the bullet on a very low setting and circle it around my clit, teasing myself. After about a minute, I begin to graze my clit, making a sort of figure-eight motion, until I come. I have to turn the vibe off right after I come, because otherwise it's just too much."
>
> —Lexi, age twenty-four

### •••SLIMLINE•••

If size matters, meaning you want something long, hard, and plastic to get off with, then Slimline vibes, which have been around since the reemergence of vibrators and will likely be around until the end of vibration, are a reliable and inexpensive start. Almost every major manufacturer makes its own version of the Slimline—some are one speed, and others offer multiple dalliances. The larger version is generally six inches long, but there are mini versions as well. They're great for providing vibration to your clit, and they're easy to hold. Plus, they give you the flexibility to play with insertion.

They generally look like a penis in shape, but not so much so in style. They're smooth plastic and come in the colors of the rainbow. They take two C batteries, and you'll notice that C batteries add more of a kick to the initial intensity of vibration. You can also check out the hard vibes by the high-end manufacturer Jimmyjane if you're looking for something insertable, although they are rather slim in the girth department. Or if music is key to your masturbatory ritual, the OhMiBod is a thin, sleek, white, hard plastic vibrator that plugs into your iPod or other MP3 player. Once it's attached, choose your tune and then let the OhMiBod help you have a rockin' good time getting off. Extra advice is to choose songs with lots of bass, because they provide a deeper vibration. Other good hard vibes are the Magnifique and the Liberté, especially if penetration is the name of your game.

> *"I like dildo vibrators because they can be used for penetration and, well, vibration. They're good for a change, or a quick fix. Like, if I'm feeling sexy in the afternoon but have somewhere to be, I can just get off quickly. And even though I like the option of putting it inside me, most often, I use it on my clit."*
>
> *—Liz, age thirty*

## SOFTER, SOFTER

### •••FUNFACTORY•••

Funfactory is a German manufacturer of quality soft toys. They make a host of softer silicone and elastomed (elastomer compound) vibes, all of which are easy to clean and are nontoxic, hypoallergenic, and odor-free (making them the antithesis of jelly rubber). A number of G-spot vibes are designed to look like animals—there's Patchy Paul (a worm), Dolly Dolphin, and Freaky Fritz (some sort of lizard/dragon). They're adorable and fun, and

Candida Royalle, the former adult-star-turned-director who pioneered the concept of films geared toward couples, was also at the forefront of the latest revolution in handheld vibrators. Her Natural Contours line of sex toys not only looks fantastic but is designed to fit nicely with the shape of most women's mounds and clitorises, and her unique aesthetic has become a staple of the adult-toy market. While her original three vibes (the Petite, the Superbe, and the Magnifique) still sell well, it's her Ultime that has gotten the most attention. A G-spot vibe that delivers vibration both inside (on

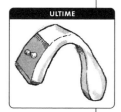

ULTIME

the spot) and on the clit (it's easy to press the vibe up against the clit while it's inside you), this hard plastic love machine is great for sexploration. With the addition of Royalle's latest creation, the Idéal, the Natural Contours line now offers eight eyegasmic options. The Idéal is the modern-day Hitachi Magic Wand. Offering the power of a plug-in, this rechargeable massager can be used on your back, neck, spine, or clit—just like the Magic Wand, only with a more logically designed handle. The first oscillating vibe in the Natural Contours collection, the Idéal offers two speeds of higher vibration, and sixty minutes of vibration per charge.

come in vibrant colors. And they'll be your best friend if they can help you find your G-spot (of course, that's only if that's a goal of yours). All of these new friends take two AA batteries.

If small is your preferred size, then the Laya is one of Funfactory's most popular designs, and, like the elegant, rechargeable, user-friendly clitoral stimulators made by the luxury Swedish company Lelo, it's a clitoral stimulator that's ergonomically designed to lie on your mound while it works on your clit. It's designed this way so you don't have to hold it in place, allowing you to enjoy a hands-free ride—well, except that you may want to control the pressure by actually holding it down there. The ergonomic shape doesn't necessarily fit every mound, but it's still a great vibe if

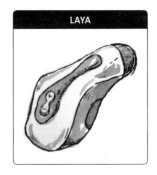

LAYA

you're looking for a small, quiet, elastomed, waterproof, variable-speed, and attractive new friend. This one takes two AAA batteries, and it can hit your G-spot if you place the smaller end inside of you!

In addition, Funfactory has teamed up with the sexpert staff at Good Vibrations to create a line of well-crafted toys that include the "splash proof" G-Swirl, a silicone version of the Nubby G (the original Nubby G is made of clear jelly rubber). Not only is the G-Swirl a multispeed soft toy with a textured shaft and a curved hook designed to hit the G-spot, but it's also made of a material I feel good about recommending to women. As an added bonus, it's got a clitoral ridge that can work on your nub while it's inside you (depending on the fit, of course). The Semirealistic, a vibrating silicone cock that only slightly resembles the real thing, comes in colors like baby blue, pale pink,

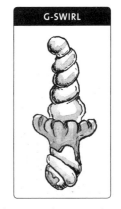

G-SWIRL

and purple; like the G-Swirl, it has a controller that's mounted at an angle, at the base of the toy, for easy attunement. Basically, you just turn the knob at the bottom of the toy to rev it up or calm it down. It's multispeed, waterproof, and curved, and takes two AA batteries.

If Funfactory's line of sex toys isn't in your budget, there are plenty of other softer options out there. Doc Johnson's line of Lucid Dream vibes are designed with transparent materials that allow you to see the inner workings of your toy. The problem with these toys is the material they're made of. I've gone to great lengths to wave a flag of caution about the dangers of phthalates in jelly rubber toys, and the Lucid Dream vibes, while aesthetically appealing, still smell like phthalates. However, they are a way more affordable option for those on a budget, and Doc Johnson is one of the large manufacturers working on ways to eradicate the bad phthalates from their material.

On a happy note, Lucid Dream vibes are good on sensation. The motor is located at the tip of the toy, which provides intense vibration to the most sensitive bits of your vagina. These are jelly rubber toys (so remember to think about using a condom with them) that get the job done and look good while doing it, even if they don't smell as good as they look.

All this is to say that even though I'm talking trash about jelly rubber, not everyone can rule out these toys, so don't feel guilty if you should want, or buy, a jelly rubber toy. I would ask, though, that if you decide to buy a jelly rubber toy, you please use a condom to keep yourself safe. If anything, do avoid the original "real" skin vibes, because, aside from being porous and containing phthalates, they're difficult to keep clean.

## PLUG IT IN OR CHARGE IT UP

Power-hungry pleasure-seekers like plug-in vibes. They are the most powerful vibes known to womankind, and the most reliable vibes on the market, generally lasting longer than most Hollywood marriages (and most other vibes). The most popular plug-in vibe is the Hitachi Magic Wand. The wand was designed as a body massager, and the truth is that it's great for sore muscles. But it's gained fame for being a popular tool for the clit, and for years now, women have discovered their orgasmic potential thanks to the

Magic Wand and other plug-in vibes. Because it's such a powerhouse of pleasure, some women need extra protection and opt to keep their panties on while getting off; others put a towel between them and the toy. The Magic Wand has two speeds, high and *holy shit,* and it's got a constant, reliable, and steady vibration. If you want more options, try the Wahl 7-in-1, another "back massager" that provides two high-speed options—along with seven heads for stimulation. The Wahl 7-in-1 store offers a version with heat, but with or without it, the Wahl 7-in-1 gives you plenty to choose from and a long cord,

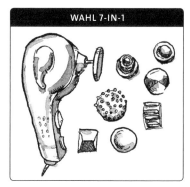

**WAHL 7-IN-1**

and it's quieter than the Magic Wand. Plus, it comes in a sexy silver color. The Eroscillator (see the "Luxury Sex" section later in this chapter) is another exceptional plug-in that comes with a long cord and different heads for your personal oscillation. Traveling with a plug-in vibe isn't always easy, especially if you're heading to a foreign country. Unless you know you've got the right converter, you might opt to leave your vibe at home when you go abroad. There are plenty of battery-operated toys that should keep you satisfied while you're away—whether it be for business or pleasure.

> *"I couldn't figure out exactly what to do to make myself come. I experimented with various finger/hand placements, with objects, and nothing. . . . Finally, I bought myself a Hitachi Magic Wand and I came. Now that was a eureka moment!"*
>
> —*Cassie, age fifty-five*

> "I use the Hitachi Magic Wand. I've tried other vibrators in the past (battery-operated ones, even the Rabbit), but once I tried the Hitachi, I wouldn't use anything else again, including my own hand! It doesn't even get me off that fast anymore, since I've been using one for several years now and it's not a new feeling. But I suppose I am lazy about coming any other way, at least when I'm alone. I also use the Hitachi a lot when I'm having sex with my female partner. We both love to incorporate it into sex."
>
> —Erica, age twenty-seven

Though plug-ins are among the most popular vibes on the market, rechargeable vibes seem to be the wave of the future. Lots of companies are making rechargeable vibes that are built to last while still being elegant, ergonomic, and higher quality. The AcuVibe is one of the oldest rechargeables, and you can find it in stores like The Sharper Image. It's the one Samantha of *Sex and the City* buys and then returns because, after six months of work, it has "failed to get her off." The AcuVibe is like the Wand, only it's got a softer, flexible head and is rechargeable. The Idéal, another spin-off of the Wand, is uniquely shaped for great back massages. In the packaging, it's the shape of a lowercase "j," complete with the point at the top (that would be the head of the massager—the part that you'd use on your clit, or wherever). Another special feature is that it oscillates like the Eroscillator, a luxury plug-in vibe that prides itself on its side-to-side movement, as opposed to actual vibration. For those who loved the old-school joysticks that you find on so many arcade games, Funfactory makes its own silicone, rechargeable, and waterproof line of vibes called the Sinnflut. Available in both regular and mini sizes, each vibe has a minijoystick at its base, allowing for quick and easy one-finger action.

Companies devised to cater to luxury-sex-toy clientele, like Lelo, Je Joue, and Emotional Bliss (you can buy their products at most retail outlets), all make rechargeable vibes too. Durex, the same company that makes condoms, has its own line of rechargeables that ranges from a Magic Wand lookalike to smaller vibes, like the Play Little Gem, that remind me of alien aircraft from the planet Vibrato. Most novelty companies make rechargeable rabbits, as well as other cute vibes, but the quality of these toys is often questionable. Almost all high-end or novelty rechargeable vibes last sixty minutes per charge, so the best way to make sure your toy is always ready to go is to clean and recharge it after each use.

> "I have a good selection of vibrators to choose from depending on my mood. My favorite is similar to the Hitachi Magic Wand, but has a metal head and a heat function. As if the vibrations weren't enough, the heat sends me to a whole new level of ecstasy. When I want to come extremely hard, I use that vibrator directly on my clit while inserting another vibrator in my pussy. My favorite combination is to use a vibrator on my clit while also having a vibrator, dildo, or fingers in my pussy while I come. I get so much more pleasure having something for my cunt to clench while I get closer and closer to orgasm and then grip hard when I finally come. Not only does it increase the intensity of my orgasm, but I imagine it must be doing wonders for my PC muscle!"
>
> —Heather, age thirty-three

**MORE BANG: DUAL-ACTION DIVAS**

Dual-action toys were created for the girl who likes a little bit of this and a little bit of that. Designed to work on both penetration and external stimulation simultaneously, dual-action toys are great if you can handle a lot of sensation.

Most dual-action toys are used for both vaginal penetration and clitoral stimulation, but you could also use the toy to stimulate your bum, or to penetrate your ass and stimulate your pussy. Dual-action toys often have a separate clitoral stimulator and penetrator; some actually come with detachable bits, and others curve in a way that allows you to hit two spots with the same toy. There are a variety of dual-action toys in the sexual universe, and since not all women are built alike, not all toys work as well for every individual. The advantage of a dual-action vibe is that if you decide you don't want it to double your pleasure, you can always use it as a regular vibe, stimulating your clit or your vagina without having to work on both.

 Japanese law used to forbid the manufacturing of phallic sex toys. So Japanese sex toy manufacturers started making vibes with clitoral stimulators in the shapes of cute little animals like rabbits and fish. And even though the shaft of some of these toys resembles a penis, you'll always find a smiling face on the tip when you turn it around.

Vibratex, the first company to bring dual-action vibes to America, makes good dual-action toys, and with most—if not all—of their products, you can rest assured that you're making a quality purchase. Their most popular toy, and really, the most popular dual-action toy ever, is the Rabbit Habit. It has a long purple shaft that looks like a penis, but not *really*, especially when you check it out up close and see that the head of the penis is actually a woman's bouffant and the backside of the toy has a woman's smiling face etched on it. It's also got a clitoral stimulator that looks like a rabbit, with vibrating ears that will send your clit into a tizzy. Plus, it has pearl beads in the shaft that rotate and provide sensation for your vaginal lips. The shaft rotates like mad if you turn it on while it's outside the body, but when it's inside you it doesn't move quite the same, especially since your vaginal muscles are clenching the shaft, not allowing it the necessary room to "breathe" (read: rotate). It's not super quiet, but that's because it has a lot going on. Plus, it's controlled by two switches, both located at the base of the toy—one

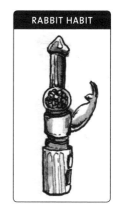

RABBIT HABIT

for the penetrative rod and one for the clitoral stimulator—and you can use one, or both at the same time. The shaft can bend, but be careful: Bending it too much, or too often, can result in the beads getting all messed up, and the toy will break.

> *"Ever since I discovered the Rabbit, it's the only way I masturbate. I love the high-speed clit action that I get from the rabbit's head, and the shaft that rolls around and rubs my G-spot. I can have orgasm after orgasm with it, and they are all mind-blowing."*
>
> —Amanda, age thirty-seven

The Rabbit Pearl is like the Rabbit Habit, except for three things: It's pink, not purple; it takes three C batteries, rather than three AA; and its operational pack is totally separate from the toy and attached by a thin, wiry cord. This makes the Rabbit Pearl more susceptible to breakage, but it's a popular option for women who enjoy using their toys not only for masturbation, but for partnered stimulation as well. With a partner you can hold the Rabbit inside you (and on your clit) while your partner lies next to you and varies the speed and the motion. Or your partner could hold the toy as you man the controls from above. Oh yeah—you'll find that sometimes the pearls in the Rabbit will get ahead of themselves and tumble over one another, which tends to throw off the toy's rotation. Gently move the pearls back into place, and you should be just fine.

Other Vibratex dual-action toys include the Twinsu. The Twinsu has pearls and a separate anal probe, which you can maneuver to your liking. You can also use the probe on your clit because, unlike the clit stimulator on the Rabbit Habit, this probe is attached to the toy by a spiral cord and therefore has flexibility in its positioning. This setup allows you more maneuverability in terms of being able to move the clit/anal probe to stimulate you in just the right places. Some people find that the cord gets in the way, but I like that it allows you more room to play. Most of the original Vibratex dual-action toys, including the original Rabbit, are made of a higher-quality soft vinyl, which means they still contain phthalates, but less phthalates than most other jelly toys. Another important note: With all Vibratex toys, make sure the switch is fully off before you put them away. Vibratex toys can be a bit sneaky like that, because, even though the toys will stop vibrating, unless you actually hear and feel an off click, the batteries might still be running. So flick until you hear and feel the click, or be doubly safe and take out the batteries, before you lay it down to rest.

One more Vibratex dual-action toy worth mentioning is the Thunder Cloud, a super-thick, soft, cyberskinlike, phthalate-free, elastomer toy that's a size queen's delight. If its giantness doesn't do it for you, it also comes complete with its very own disco-light system. Yes, that's right: At full speed it continuously flashes red, blue, and green—just in case you needed another reason to buy something so outrageously big, soft, and white. You don't have to worry about pearls with this one (there are none), and while elastomer is still porous, it's a health-conscious alternative for those with latex allergies, or for those of us who are supportive of phthalate-free toys that still offer a soft, dual-action option.

The good news is that Vibratex is now making many of their newer toys with latex- and phthalate-free elastomer, including an updated version of the Rabbit. While you can still buy the original soft-vinyl Rabbit Habit, this newest version is called the Elastomer Rabbit Habit. It's been updated a bit in terms of design. The clitoral rabbit portion is more angled for better clit contact, and the pearls (there are fewer of them) are redesigned to rotate more consistently than they do in the original.

Another of these newer toys, the Vibratex Original Deluxe Japanese Butterfly Vibrator, looks more like a robot bug than a butterfly, really. It's made of elastomer and requires three AA batteries. It's shaped like all of Vibratex's dual-action vibes, but its body has larger pearls and its head has ridges, both of which feel great upon entry. Unlike the Rabbit, the "butterfly" clit stimulator is located closer to the head of the toy (what most women would describe as "a better position"), and its wings are great for tickling the labia. Plus, the vibrating clit part is right in the center of the "vaginally inspiring" pearls, which is great for women who don't want to have to insert the toy as far back as their cervix in order to stimulate their clit. And, unlike in older Vibratex toys, the controller is two rotating dials, instead of up and down switches. As an added bonus, it has another separate on-off switch, a smart design response to that problem of the toy's seeming to be off when it's really still running.

Funfactory makes a host of silicone, dual-action toys, too. All part of the Twist 'n' Shake series, each of these vibes has rotating pearls in the center of its shaft and a separate stimulator for the clit. They're controlled at the base with separate switches—one for "twist" and one for "shake"—and all of them are made of nonporous material. The Paul and Paulina vibe looks like a pair of worms; Mary Mermaid has a beautiful, feminine, mermaid-style shaft; and Sally Sea is a sea lioness. All take four AA batteries.

If dual action sounds like too much for you, fear not—there are some less complicated options that don't require separate switches or stimulators to help you achieve that combination orgasm. As mentioned earlier, toys such as the Ultime and the Rock-Chick are curved in a shape that resembles the letter U, and provide vaginal stimulation (upon insertion) and clitoral stimulation (when you press the outer part of the toy into your best bud). You can use the toy to rock back and forth, which is what inspired the latter's name. The Ultime is made of hard blue plastic; the Rock-Chick is purple medical-grade silicone. The silicone option is more expensive, but both are designed with the same intention—to hit your G-spot while vibrating your clit. The Rock-Chick is a one-speed toy, though the newest models come complete with a longer, stronger RO 80-millimeter vibrating bullet that's powered by N-type LR1 alkaline batteries (the battery looks like a AA battery that's been cut in half). The Ultime has three speeds and takes two AA batteries.

Dual-action toys that have a separate clitoral stimulator and vaginal penetrator don't work for everybody. In fact, the biggest complaint about these toys is that they don't fit certain women's bodies. It's important to remember that if you purchase a toy like this and you're not wowed by it, nothing is wrong with you. No toy works the same for every woman.

 **ACTION! ACTION! ACTION!**

If dual action seems so passé and you're still looking for more bang for your bottom, triple-action vibrators work your pussy, your clit, and your anus. Loveologist Dr. Ava Cadell invented what she calls her TriGasm: The butt plug is detachable in order to fit any body type, and the controls give you eight different speeds, vibrations, and pulsations. While it's not the most aesthetically pleasing vibe out there (the long shaft has a pointy tip that made me feel like running when I first saw it), Dr. Cadell put a lot of time and research into her invention, and it's the only triple-action toy I've seen that has so many pulsation/vibration options—and a removable butt plug so that you don't have to use it on the days when you don't feel like being all filled up. The unfortunate thing is that the TriGasm is vinyl and porous, which means you should put a condom on the parts that you insert inside you. It takes four AA batteries.

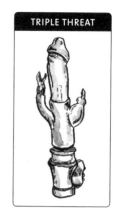

**TRIPLE THREAT**

There are lots of other inexpensive triple-action vibes out there, like the Triple Threat and the Amour. These vibes offer triple stimulation without any removable/adjustable bits. The Triple Threat has a longer tail, which makes it easier to hit your bum, while the Amour has a little nub that's designed to hit your ass (but you have to penetrate pretty deeply to get there). And, while less expensive than the TriGasm, neither of these options is as clever in design. Still, they have dials to control the intensity. One dial controls the shaft and the other works the clit/anal stimulators. Both take four AA batteries and should be used with a condom as well.

 **LUXURY SEX**

In the past few years a number of companies have sprung up with the sheer determination and desire to make elegant, safe, and reliable vibrating sex toys. These companies include Elemental Pleasures, Emotional Bliss, Eroscillator, Je Joue, Jimmyjane, Lelo, and Twisted Products. The biggest turnoff about the toys is their high prices, but once you decide to take the plunge and get your hands (and clit) on one of these vibes, you will be totally turned on.

## ELEMENTAL PLEASURES

Elemental Pleasures makes a super-expensive set of vibes called Le Tigre, Panthère, and Léopard ($395 each). They come in materials like stainless steel (Léopard) and aircraft-grade aluminum (Le Tigre, Panthère), and are designed in the United States by mechanical engineers who once worked on the parts of commercial airplanes. All of the $395 vibes come complete with a velvet-lined storage box, lock, and key, and with three separate heads to choose from, depending on the speed you want: high, medium, or low. They're heavy, hot tub–proof, and boilable, and they provide fantastic vibration to the bits that need it most. They require three lithium CR123 batteries because they have 50 percent more energy-storage capacity than regular AAs, which makes replacing them a challenge—and, yes, a bit more expensive. If you're looking for the cheapest of their models, you can get the Single Kit with one high-speed head for $275 (you save $120 by not getting the two additional heads). If you're looking for the most expensive, Le Lynx is made of medical-grade titanium, comes with the same three tips, and costs a whopping $595. At least it comes with a one-year limited warranty.

## EMOTIONAL BLISS

Emotional Bliss toys are designed in the United Kingdom, and, while they have a sterile, old-fashioned aesthetic to them, the company spent three years researching, and a total of five years developing, vibes that women

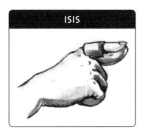

ISIS

would be comfortable using. The results of all that hard work are five vibes: two finger vibes (the Isis, $72, and Chandra, $82) and three larger vibes (the Femblossom, Jasmine, and Womolia, $132 each) that are designed with unique shapes and provide different sensations to the clit and vulva.

The Femblossom is ideal for the entire vulva; the Jasmine is designed for maximum clit stimulation and has added "stipples," tiny bumps on the tip of the vibe to offer your clit an extra dose of sensation; and the Womolia is created to hit the "orgasmic platform," which combines stimulation of the first two inches inside the vagina and the external arousal of the clit. All three vibes now have a new, more powerful motor with nine different functions (the finger vibes still have only one speed, one function). The two finger vibes have three different bands, so they'll fit on thin and thick fingers. When fully charged (twelve hours later), these vibes last anywhere between one and two hours.

## EROSCILLATOR

The Eroscillator is the only sex product endorsed by Dr. Ruth, which kind of dates it; regardless, this is one vibrator you won't regret buying. Ever. Imagine taking your electric toothbrush and having it all tricked out with the best sex accessories you could possibly hope for, and that's what you get with the Eroscillator. Instead of the shallow vibration provided by most other vibrating sex toys, this one oscillates 3,600 times per minute. That means it actually moves in an individual side-to-side motion, rather than a quick back-and-forth vibrating one. The team at Advanced Response Corporation (parent company of the folks who make the Eroscillator) truly believe that research is

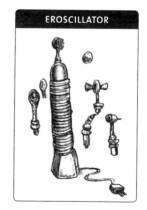

EROSCILLATOR

worth every penny. (They spent $2 million and seven years on research, and each vibe comes with a one-year warranty.) Manufactured in Switzerland, this plug-in vibrator is all about providing the best stimulation possible, and trust me, it doesn't disappoint. It's got three speeds, an assortment of heads (called "flabbergasmic attachments"), and a plug with a very, very long cord. It's quiet enough that if you're using it alone in your bedroom, you'll be the only one who knows. You can buy a basic or ultimate combo package, and prices range from $127.95 to $240.90.

## JE JOUE

Je Joue looks more like the by-product of a cell phone that mated with a remote control than like a standard vibrator, and that's because this vibe is anything but standard. A pretty, purple rechargeable toy with excellent packaging, it's the must-have vibe for any number-one fan of long foreplay sessions. It comes with three elastomer pads that you actually slip over the hard plastic nub on the underside of the toy (the side you'll use on your clit). Use some lube on your clit (Je Joue includes its own samples of silicone lube with your purchase) and let Je Joue do its thing. It comes with ten "grooves," which are preprogrammed patterns designed to get you off in a variety of quivers, tickles, and turns. When you turn on the vibe, you get a number of options to choose from, like "Quickie" (great if all you've got is five minutes to get off, 'cause this one comes to a climax that quick) and "Cleaner," which does my favorite full-circle motion (think of the head cleaner used for cassettes and VHS tapes). All ten grooves are programmed to do different up-and-down, side-to-side, pulsing, quivering, and round-and-round motions. It's not actual music, but it's as close as you're going to get to making your own orgasmic composition. And if you find yourself in the middle of the best dance ever, you can hit the "Don't Stop" button on the front of the vibe to ensure that you'll keep going with the flow. Plus, by installing the PleasureWare software it comes with, you can download different tracks (up to ten of your own) that allow you to create your own combination of vibes to get off to. And, like with file-sharing, you can share them in the Je Joue community. Plus, it includes a velour carrying case, a

USB cable (for downloading to your Je Joue), and instructions. It's expensive ($290), but if you're a geek, or a girl who loves them, then this is the smartest sex toy around.

## JIMMYJANE

Now, if you love the Pocket Rocket because it's small, one-speed, and easy to use, but you'd rather pamper yourself for your pleasure, then you'll love Jimmyjane's Little Something series. All the vibes in the Little Something series have replaceable motors, which means they will last a lifetime, or as long as you're willing to replace the motor for $35 a pop. They take one AA battery, and they're totally waterproof. These vibes come in your choice of gold ($275), steel ($195), or platinum ($395), which allows you to warm them up or cool them down—something you can't do with plastic. And they're relatively quiet, but not silent.

If you like your vibes to pop visually, Little Chroma is the colorful counterpart of Little Something. Same vibe, just with an added splash of color. Little Chroma, made of high-quality anodized aluminum ($165), comes in olive, orange, magenta, and red. Jimmyjane's latest vibe is the Form 6 ($175), which comes with a rechargeable lithium-ion battery and six digital modes. It's designed to fit in your hand and conform to your body. Made of medical-grade plum or green silicone, as well as stainless steel, it's got two motors and you can use either end of the toy for stimulation.

## LELO

Lelo makes some of the prettiest vibes on the market. This Swedish company has worked hard to make products that not only look feminine, sleek, and sensual, but feel mighty fine, too. All Lelo toys are rechargeable, including the Iris ($134), the Nea ($89), and the Lily ($129). The Iris has two individually placed vibrating motors that operate together, or alone, to provide you with the stimulation (and/or pulsation) you need to get off. It looks like a budding flower or a peeled banana, depending on your mood, and it comes in pale pink or baby blue, with just enough of an angle at the tip to hit the right places. The Nea and Lily are smaller clitoral stimulators, the former having a porcelainlike finish, the latter made of elastomer. Both are curved for easy handling, and all of Lelo's vibes really are as quiet as they say they are.

## THE CONE (TWISTED PRODUCTS)

Twisted Products's Cone looks like a mini-me version of the kind of cone you'd see in traffic (except it's pink). The Cone is a soft, silicone, hands-free, powerful vibrating toy that allows you to get off clitorally while doing other things, like playing video games or lying on your tummy and reading a book of erotica. It's got a powerful motor and sixteen different functions, and

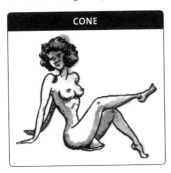

there are enough interesting options to keep you entertained for a while. If you're looking for something totally unique, you can't find a more interestingly shaped toy. Its negatives are its bulk and weight, the fact that it takes three C batteries, and its loud sound—in one of the more intense vibratory positions, I thought there was a single-engine plane flying overhead, and then I realized it was only my toy. But the weight encourages you to get clever with positions, like placing it up on the wall and backing into it, squatting on top of it, or sitting with your legs wrapped around it while you watch TV. You can put the tip of the Cone inside you, but really it's for vibrating your outside areas, and it does so quite nicely. Plus, how many toys come with instructions in twenty-four languages?

**VIBING WITH YOUR PARTNER**

I love vibrators because they helped me learn to orgasm. If you've never had an orgasm (and if you have to think about whether you have, then odds are you haven't), or if you want to get there with less work, then the vibrator is, for many, a quick fix. A vibrator can teach you about places on your own body you never thought about touching, and it can help you take charge of your orgasms.

Of course, there are some things a vibrator can't do, like replace your hands, your partner, or your fuck buddy. A vibrator doesn't cuddle, kiss, or communicate, and it won't ever be able to tell you how beautiful and amazing you are, even if it can make you feel pretty and confident. So when, or if, your partner expresses concern over the bond between you and your toy, remind them that a vibrator is there to help you explore your sexual pleasure. If you feel comfortable, introduce your partner to the wonderful world of vibration and explore it together. They may be quite surprised by just how much they like it as well.

Remember, a vibrator is only one of the ways to experience pleasure. So enjoy its sensations but experiment with other sex toys, and forms of communication, as well. There are a whole lot of ways to have sex, and trying as many of them as you feel comfortable with will allow you to open yourself up to a larger universe of sexual exploration, regardless of how much, or how often, you get your buzz on.

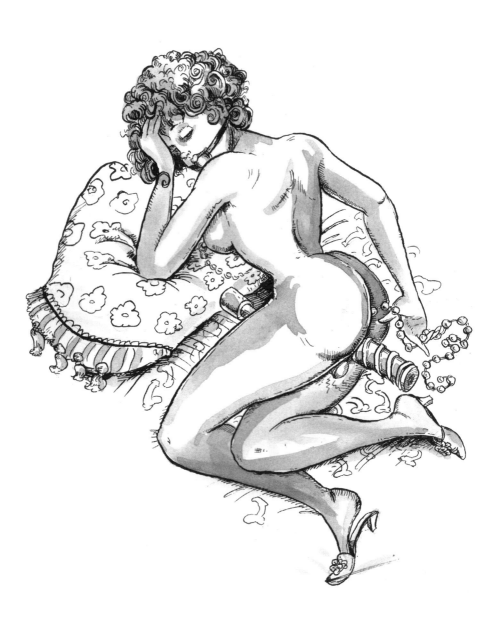

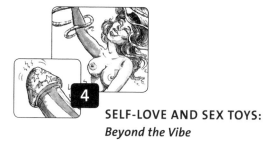

## SELF-LOVE AND SEX TOYS:
### Beyond the Vibe

THERE'S NO GOLDEN RULE THAT SAYS how to masturbate, or what you must use to get the job done. Lots of women go their whole lives without flicking anything other than a finger, but with so many new sex toys manufactured each year, it's no secret that a little help can go a long way.

> "Since I moved back home, my bag of sex toys is in storage, so now, when I get the chance (read: when my mom isn't home), I use an electric razor with the blade taken out. It's fine, but it sure ain't my Magic Wand."
>
> —Kiley, age twenty-seven

What is a sex toy? A sex toy is anything that can be used for sexual pleasure. It's an object that's used during sex or masturbation to tune in and turn on various parts of your body. A sex toy excites your body in places like your clit, your nipples, your vulva, your skin, your brain, and your ass. It can be used for penetration or external stimulation. It heightens your senses, builds your arousal, and enhances sexual activity. If a vibrator is the first or only thing that pops into your head when you think about sex toys, you're not alone. However, women were playing with toys long before the invention of batteries and electrical outlets. Sex toys don't have to be "sex toys" at all; in fact, for some women a sex toy is whatever is around when she needs it most. For instance, one woman's sex toy might be another woman's appliance (a cell phone or the washing machine, for instance), but most sex toys are bought at a sex shop, drugstore, or gadget shop.

When it comes to masturbation, sex toys can take self-pleasure to a whole new level. They can be placed inside or on your body; they can help you focus attention on places you might not otherwise reach. When they're used inside the vagina or the butt, they make it easier to access your G-spot. They also feel good at the very entrance of your pussy, because the entrance of the vagina is more sensitive than the inside. And they're great either as a warm-up or to help you cross the finish line.

> "I like sex toys because using them often leads to stronger orgasms than I can produce with my hands or my pillows. I've hurt my wrists pretty badly a couple of times from masturbating, so they prevent that from happening, too!"
>
> —Blythe, age thirty-two

 **THINGS THAT MAKE YOU GO *OOOH!***

When it comes to sex toys for self-pleasure, women like to use all different kinds of things: dildos, vibrators, butt plugs, nipple clamps, lube, feathers, and gags. Sex toys are easy to use alone or with a partner; they're good for heightening sensations during any kind of stimulation.

 Sexual privacy is not something you can take for granted down South. According to an Alabama statute, it is "unlawful for any person to knowingly distribute . . . any obscene material or any device designed or marketed as useful primarily for the stimulation of human genital organs."[1]

## DILDOS

Back in the day, there was no silicone or soft vinyl, no hard plastic or jelly rubber. When the Chinese first made dildos, they were cut out of wood, jade, ivory, and bronze.[2] In different parts of the world, dildos were also made out of other stones and leather, and the *Kama Sutra* refers to dildos made of wood and reed. Artifacts that resemble dildos have been found in Upper Paleolithic art from more than thirty thousand years ago.[3]

 The once-bustling city of Miletus in ancient Greece was a thriving dildo manufacturer, and ancient Greek women would go there to buy handmade large, small, fat, slim, and carved *olisbos* for personal enjoyment.[4]

---

### TOYS FOR TWATS

The vagina is approximately six inches long in an aroused state. The average-size dildo is the same as the average-size penis (approximately five and a half inches), but there are so many sizes and shapes that "average" is just one of many choices. You can get ones as long as fourteen inches and others as short as one or two. Any size you want is basically out there for the taking, but it's the first third of the vagina that's the most sensitive, so finding something that will satisfy your entrance is usually more important than finding something to satisfy your cervix.

---

So, what is a dildo? A dildo is a nonvibrating, straight or curved object that you use inside your vagina or butt. It can be long or short, thick or thin, red or white, soft or hard. The most popular materials for dildos include jelly rubber, silicone, cyberskin, and glass. Some dildos stick out straight, others curve toward the sky, and others are as twisty as San Francisco's famed Lombard Street.

Lots of objects can be considered dildos; it all depends on how loose your definition of the word is. Things like fruits, vegetables, broomsticks, pencils, and Q-tips have all been used for that express purpose. It's a matter of personal taste—and sometimes desperation—when it comes to getting the job done. While you won't find fruits and veggies (or other household gadgets, for that matter) for sale at a local sex emporium, you will find, among other toys, a rainbowlike array of dildos, in all colors and skin tones. Some glitter and some shine. Some will remind you of a penis from your past (or possibly your present), and still others will look like abstract works of art. A dildo can be the size of your middle finger, or long and wide, like a canister of tennis balls. It can be curved or straight, chunky or slender, or a combination of any of the above. It can have a flared base, meaning that the bottom part is wider than the top, which not only helps it stand up straight, but allows it to be used for butt stuff as well. Others have no base at all, and still others have an easy-to-grip endpiece that works like a handle. When shopping for a dildo, you want to consider both length and girth. Length is easily determined from the tip to the base, but girth is more about the widest point on the toy, which isn't necessarily a measure of the size of the entire toy.

> "For a long time I used a pencil to rub my clit because I liked having something from outside my body touching me. It felt more like someone else that way. Now and then I have a strong desire to have something inside my vagina. I've tried a variety of things: medicine bottles, the handles of kitchen utensils, basically anything that wouldn't break or leave residue in me. If it's in my house, I've probably tried it!"
>
> —Laura, age forty-one

A dildo can give you the same feelings you get from partnered sex. It can make you feel satiated and stuffed. It can apply additional pressure to your special spots. It can move inside you the way a partner does, add additional stimulation to your bum, or hit the places your fingers can't. Whatever your reasons for liking dildos, when shopping for one the most important question to ask yourself is, *What do I want to stick inside of me?* Then think about the girth. More than length, thickness or thinness will make all the difference.

Some of the nicest dildos are a lot more expensive than, say, a household gadget like a flashlight or a broomstick, but these dildos not only are safer and sturdier, they're also built to last. Still, if you decide to try something around the house, even something disposable like a zucchini, make sure that you take the time to use it correctly. Any vegetables should be used with their skins on, and only after they've been wrapped in a condom. Any other household appliances should be protected so that you don't harm yourself or make the toy unsanitary for its actual created use. Truthfully, buying a dildo that's meant to be used as a sex toy is your best and smartest bet, but sometimes, and in certain circumstances, it's not an option.

Now, if you do buy a dildo, you want to invest wisely. Find something that won't bore you over time (or be prepared to buy another dildo once that happens), and find one that you'll enjoy using when you crave that full-up feeling.

## BUTT STUFF

In the Victorian era, one European doctor advised his male patients to insert a wooden egg up their bums to help decrease the loss of semen. Even though this is one of the oldest recorded stories of butt plug usage in Western civilization, anal accoutrements have definitely been around since long before that.[5] The more popular butt plugs you find today are different from the ones prescribed by the wooden egg–loving doctor, since most of them have flared bases. A flared base is like a safety belt, stopping the toy from moving all over the place, and preventing it from sliding up into your bum. A flared base means that the bottom of the toy extends wider than

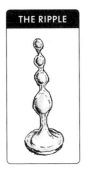

**THE RIPPLE**

the body of the toy, and therefore acts like a stopper, preventing the toy from slipping up into the deep space of Uranus, from which it might otherwise need to be surgically removed.

Plugs are designed to stuff you up—like a holiday meal, only without the tummyaches, the sleepiness, or the added calories. Butt plugs stimulate your bum but can also hit your G-spot, and since your anal passage is also your vagina's next-door neighbor (with walls as thin as the walls in a New York City high-rise) you can definitely hit one spot by entering the other. Anal play is also a good way to stimulate the fourchette (where the inner lips meet at the base of the vagina) and other sensitive bits and pieces that surround the ass.

If you've never played with your bum before and want to give it a try, don't shy away from the experience. Start in the shower, when you're all lathered up and sudsy. Gently rub your finger around the rim of your bum, and massage the area with small finger circles. After you feel relaxed, slowly press the tip of your soapy finger up into your anus. Contract and release the muscles to your butt, and notice the sensations. Press around. See what works for you and what doesn't.

**TIP** If you don't want to hold the dildo inside of you, try stuffing a pair of shorts or pants with pillows or towels. Place the dildo in the zipper part of the shorts and zip it up for stability. If your clothes don't have a zipper, or the dildo won't stay in place, buy a harness (you can purchase one at any sex shop) and strap it onto your stuffed bottoms. Experiment with the angle and position of your stuffed shorts. And then enjoy the ride.

When the urge hits outside the shower, go for it, girl, but don't underestimate the value of lubrication. Our vaginas self-lubricate, but our bums will not. So, before you go in with the tip of your finger or any other toy, make sure that there's lube in your butt, and on whatever it is you're planning on inserting into you. Once inside, gently stretch out your sphincter muscles. This will relax them and give them a nice Jane Fonda–esque warm-up. When you feel confident that you can handle more, it's time for your toy.

**TIP** Never use a toy up your bum without a condom (unless it's boilable). If you do, make sure that the toy you use in your tush is a toy that you use *only* in your tush.

Sure, you could shove a dildo (one with a base, please) into your rear entry, but when it comes to your ass, a butt plug is still a good first bet. Like dildos, butt plugs can be bumpy, straight, curved, thick, or thin. A butt plug is often designed to stay put, meaning that once it's in, it's in, and you can then focus on other areas of your personal topography. To use a butt plug, get yourself going and then slowly begin to insert the well-lubed plug up your bum. Oh—if you get the feeling that you have to go to the bathroom once you start to clog your drain, fear not. Once a plug, or any other object, is placed inside your bum, you can get that sense of urgency that sometimes surrounds the feeling of having to poop. But it's more likely than not that you don't have to, unless you had to go before you began. In that case, you shouldn't have ignored nature's call. But having something inside you can make you feel like you have to go when you really don't. Just breathe. Relax. Chill out. Hang out with the toy until you feel ready to move forward. And once that have-to-go feeling subsides, slowly make your way farther in. The keys to getting over that initial reaction are relaxation, breathing, and patience.

If a butt plug isn't your style, you can try anal beads (you can use these in your pussy, too, but not the same pair that you use in your butt). While they're great to wear during masturbation, they're even more fun to pull out as you cross the finish line. Anal beads are generally a series of smooth, round balls or beads that are separated by a small nylon string, or by small

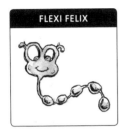

FLEXI FELIX

sections of silicone or jelly rubber. The latter is the more sanitary option because nylon strings get dirty and can't really be cleaned. Some come in a string of equal-size beads, while others get progressively larger toward the tail end of the toy. To use anal beads, push that first smaller ball in, and then, after you're used to how it feels, get those remaining beads up there. You'll notice that lots of anal beads have a specific front and back side, and that the end of the toy has either a ring or some other handlelike shape for you to grip when you're ready to remove the toy from your body. When you're ready to peak, pull the beads straight out of your bum for a uniquely contractional experience. *And don't forget lube!*

Dildos and vibrators are also great for the bum, but you want to make sure that they're going to be long enough to not accidentally slip out of your grasp, or that they have a larger base than shaft for extra protection. And you don't want to share a toy that you use in your ass with other parts of your body, or other people, unless you can sterilize the toy, or unless you are obsessively adamant about putting a condom over that sucker every time you use it. The bacteria from your ass can cause funky things to happen in your vagina, and you never want to go from back to front with the same toy in the same session.

You can insert a dildo or butt plug into your bum at any time during the buildup, but it will usually feel nicer if you wait until you're really excited to take it all in. That means you want to be aroused, and you want to want it in you. You want to want it in you so bad, you can't imagine why it's not already there. And then, when you feel like the time is right, you want to make sure to love your toy with lube. After the toy is slick, you can slowly, or quickly, depending on your preference and level of experience, insert it inside yourself. You might want to start by massaging around the rim, with either your finger or a finger vibe like the Fukuoko 9000.

> "I basically use a form of dildo these days. My favorites are the anal bead toys, but I use them in my pussy instead of in my ass. If they're the long, bendable kind then I might put one side up my pussy, and the other up my ass. I'm not much into vibration, because I swear I have seen fools get dependent on that shit. I've had friends swear they couldn't get off unless it's with a vibrator. I think they're just blocked, y'know, like writer's block, only this is orgasm block."
>
> —Cocacolachola, age twenty-nine

Now, if you're feeling like you want an abundance of sextasy overload, you can also go in for double penetration. Double penetration entails masturbating simultaneously with a dildo and butt plug, in your pussy and anus. While you do this you can still massage your clit with a finger or vibe. It's great for bringing you over the edge!

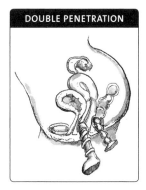

**DOUBLE PENETRATION**

Double penetration requires arousal, so you want to start by turning yourself on in your most erogenous and sensitive places. Lying on your back, rub around your clit with a finger or two, sliding your pointer finger into your pussy when you feel like it and then using your natural wetness to massage your clit again and again. If you think you're going to have an orgasm, or at any point when you're definitively and totally turned on, stop what you're doing to prolong your experience. Squeeze your breasts, rub your thighs, do whatever you like to do to keep yourself going (but stop yourself from coming). Of course you could also have an orgasm at any point and then start over again!

Next, take a dildo and begin to move it in and out of your moist vagina (if you need lube to make yourself wet, make sure to use some). Continue to do that until you feel like you want to take some more in, and then grab a lubed butt plug and work it around the entrance of your bum. Massage

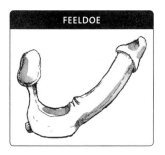

FEELDOE

your clit while you do this so that you're relaxed even more, and then slowly insert the plug into your ass. Once it's in there as far as it can go—meaning that the flared base is resting nicely on or in between your butt cheeks—bring your attention back to your front side and return that dildo to its rightful place in your pussy. Use one hand to maneuver the dildo as it penetrates your vagina, and use the other hand to rub your clit. Squeeze your ass muscles around the butt toy, and your PC muscle around the dildo, and continue to fuck yourself with one hand while you flick yourself off with the other. This will allow you to experience the fullest extent of solo fornication possible.

> "When I masturbate I like using double dildos: one in my vagina and one in my ass, and then I play with my clit. I like that it's sort of dirty, and it makes me come twice as hard."

—Natasha, age twenty-three

## NIPPLE CLAMPS

A lot of women experience pleasure in having their nipples pinched, twisted, or suckled during partnered sex play, so why not find another way to stimulate those suckers when you're alone and engorged? Nipple clamps make a fun addition to solo sex, especially for those who take some pleasure in pain. It's definitely sexy to tweak your tits as you twiddle your twat, and nipple clamps are the perfect sexessory to help you do just that. Clamps can feel sensationally sweet or brutally beautiful, and they will draw additional pinching, biting, and tugging attention to your upper half while you *hand*-le your lower self.

Even though clothespins can work as a substitute for store-bought clampage, as a beginner you'll probably want to find clamps that allow you to adjust your pleasure/pain threshold. When you're ready to invest in your first pair of clamps, you'll notice that most are attached together by a chain, and that there are some clamps that even vibrate (they're generally made of lots of plastic bits and take watch batteries). Lots of the non-vibrating metal nipple clamps have black vinyl, padded tips that act as a form of protection between your skin and the toy. These tips aren't tightly attached to the clamps and therefore often fall off, so it's a good idea to Krazy Glue the vinyl pads onto the clamp before you ever use them. This way you'll always have the softer, padded tip as protection between you and the clamp. Regardless of what clamps you choose (basic beginner or the more advanced metal shenanigans), you'll definitely feel the clamp, especially since you'll experience a surge of sharp awareness around your nipples once you set them in place. This initial sensation will subside rather quickly, however, the longer the clamps stay on, the more it'll hurt to come off. Remember that your pain threshold can change depending on where you're at in your cycle, and you shouldn't leave clamps in place for more than twenty minutes at a time.

> "I honestly don't know what tits and nipples are for (recreationally) except pinching and tugging. Clamps help take care of that and leave your hands free for other fun! I love the clovers because they get tighter when you pull on them (yum), instead of others that start out extra snug and need to be loosened for any pressure variation. Clovers are also fun for other tender bits that love pressure and attention."
>
> —C. J., age thirty

Nipple clamps aren't used only on nipples. If you'd like a good pinch below the belt, you can use clamps to open up your labia, or even place one on your clit. You can use clamps to expose more of your vulva, or as punishment for being a "naughty" girl. Whatever you choose to do with your clamps, enjoy the dual sensations of pleasure and pain.

### BEN WA BALLS

Originating in ancient Japan, Ben Wa balls (which weren't called Ben Wa balls back then) are tiny, marblelike metal balls used for both stimulation and vaginal strengthening. Back in the day they were made of either metal or ivory, and although Ben Wa balls still exist today (they're generally gold plated), they aren't as popular as they once were.[6] Since many women aren't comfortable with placing two tiny metal balls inside their vaginas, duotone balls, like Funfactory's Smartballs, are the modern girl's Ben Wa. These colorful, silicone-coated round balls are actually four balls, not two. On the inside of each silicone ball is another metal ball, and this smaller, harder ball floats freely inside the larger, hollow silicone-encased

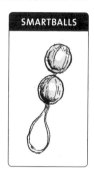

**SMARTBALLS**

sphere. The two larger silicone balls are then attached together by a small, coated cord. Smartballs are not extra large by any means, but they are larger than traditional Ben Wa balls. This added girth actually provides some women with more peace of mind when they place the balls up their birth canals, although, rest assured, nothing can get lost inside your vagina. Smartballs are light and quiet, and a hair smaller in diameter than your standard-size golf ball, and there's even a tamponlike string at the bottom for easy pullout. You basically insert one ball inside yourself and then the other, and they stay put vaginally, just like that.

> "When I masturbate with Smartballs, I sometimes tug on the string with one hand so that the lower ball rubs against my G-spot. The balls have slight indentations scored on their sides, so it's entirely possible that these grooves give extra friction. I always concentrate on the muscles in my pussy, tightening and releasing them, sucking them in and pooching them out. I have found that as I wear them more frequently I have much better control of my muscles, can clench them much harder, and get more excited with my pussy muscle play."
>
> —Chelsea Summers, age forty-four

Duotone balls are great to keep in your vagina as you masturbate your clit, and they're also great to walk around with in you, to help strengthen your PC muscle. The only warning: Until you have really strong pelvic-floor muscles, make sure to wear panties while using these balls. If you're just walking around with them in you, over time they can start to slip out of your slit, and that can create an embarrassing situation if you happen to be out shopping in a skirt.

## PUMP UP THE VOLUME

A clit pump is like the cherry on top of a sundae: unnecessary, but an added extra. Clit pumping isn't for everyone, but for those of you interested in pumping up, use lube to form a good seal between yourself and the toy. All pumps are designed with a little cap, or tube, that you place over the clitoris, which in turn is attached to another, thinner tube and a pump. Squeezing the pump creates the vacuum that then engorges your clit with blood. For women who pump, the visual of an enlarged clitoris is exciting, and the sensations that come about from feeling your ripe, sensitive pearl can send shivers up and down your spine. Clit pumps should not be used for more than a few minutes at a time, and they can be used on the nipples, too!

## BONDAGE FOR ONE

If kink really turns you on, then there's no reason not to get kinky with your bad self. Placing a blindfold over your eyes while you masturbate can help to block outside thoughts and allow you to go into a deep, dark fantasy. Want to shut yourself up? Try a ball gag, a rubber or silicone sphere that's attached to a leather or plastic strap. The strap runs through the center portion of the ball, and then you place the ball part in your mouth to muffle your sounds. People who enjoy ball gags like the look, feel, and fantasy associated with using one, even though these fantasies are generally not politically correct.

When using a ball gag, place the ball in your mouth, behind your teeth, and secure the strap around your head. The actual balls vary in size, but larger ball gags are not safe, especially since they can cause damage to your jaw. So either go with a small ball gag or try a bit gag, an alternative that's a "bit" more comfortable for the wearer. Oh, and if you start to drool, you probably won't be able to stop, but that's part of the ball gag's appeal. You can also make your own over-the-mouth gag in the form of a scarf or bandanna, which will be a lot easier on your jaw. Just pull the scarf over your mouth and tie it around at the back of your head. Again, this is great if you're into fantasy role-playing—either with yourself or a partner—and it allows you to really get into a very different headspace.

 ## SEX TOYS: WHAT, NO INSTRUCTIONS?

Sex toys don't usually come with instructions for proper handling. We're lucky that large manufacturers tell us what batteries to buy to operate any vibrating purchase, but that's often as far as they'll go to help you use their products. Perhaps most of them think that once it's in you, or rubbing up against you, you'll know what to do with it—and for the most part, you will. Soon enough you'll figure out what feels good and what doesn't, and you'll take it from there. Most insertable sex toys are fairly basic in how they operate. The toy can remain in place inside you, or move in and out of you, or tease you and rub up against you before being popped indoors.

What can help make you more comfortable in your self-discovery process is position. Will you be sitting up or lying down? Will you be on your back, on your belly, or maybe on your side? Will you use pillows for comfort or for propping yourself up to better hit your favorite places? Will you be close to a mirror so you can watch some of your own hot girl-on-toy action? Playing with yourself in front of a mirror is a fantastic way to get in touch with your own body because it allows you to watch your personal transformation from arousal to orgasm. Decisions! Decisions!

These are things you'll have to figure out once you select the toys you want to play with. There's no one way to go at it, no one toy to use, no one way to feel. Sex toys are there for your pleasure, so use only the ones that bring you joy. Pure, unbelievable, ecstatically orgasmic joy—yeah, that's the ticket!

 ## MASTURBATION MATERIAL

We're living in a material world, and there are lots of materials out there, girl. There are soft materials and hard materials, squishy types and smooth ones, porous and nonporous plastics, as well as silicones, acrylics, and heavy metals. Whatever you decide to rock out with, when you're shopping for your pleasure, material matters.

### JELLY RUBBER

While jelly rubber toys are the least expensive, they also contain phthalates (a chemical used to soften PVC), and you should therefore consider their long-term effects on your body. The truth is, they smell pretty funky, and in 2004 the European Union started to phase out phthalates from children's toys because of the dangers associated with young tykes putting these chemically infested toys in their mouths.[7] However, if you like how these toys feel, or if money matters, it's not a bad idea to put a condom on your jelly rubber toy before you play with it. It'll keep you protected and make the toy easier to clean. But no matter how clean you keep it, you'll notice a slight to severe discoloration over the course of time, because jelly rubber is an inexpensive material and discoloration is just a fact of life when it comes to choosing, and using, this product.

## HARD PLASTIC

Hard plastic is great for transmitting vibrati
side you. It all depends on what you like, of cou
of phthalates, even though they sometimes ha
lect bacteria or cause irritation. They're also gre
long as you're okay with the fact that there's no

## SILICONE

Silicone is softer than hard plastic, but not often as soft as some jelly rubber. Still, it's soft enough, and it's such a durable, long-lasting material that,
in my opinion, it's the best soft material for your box. It's not porous, which

means bacteria won't make a home in your toy, and
it comes in many colors, just like Joseph's amazing
Technicolor dreamcoat (including colors that glitter).
Silicone is also durable, and it can retain heat or cold,
depending on what temperature you want your toy
to be. To clean it, you can boil it or wash it with the
dishes (top rack only). If you're going to buy silicone,
make sure it's 100 percent silicone, because otherwise you're still getting less than you bargained for,

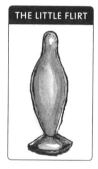

**THE LITTLE FLIRT**

meaning your toy doesn't have the same benefits (nonporous, boilable,
hygienic), and isn't as "safe," as a pure silicone product. Don't boil silicone
toys that vibrate, unless you can remove the vibrating bits. And avoid using
silicone lubes with silicone toys, because they don't react well together.

"There was a huge lack of knowledge about silicone when I decided to start Tantus, Inc. The buying public didn't know about it—that it's a hypoallergenic, hygienic material that you can boil, bleach, wash in your dishwasher, and put in an autoclave. My intention was to make a product that was more femme, and one that could last a lifetime. It was a selfish product. I made it for me, and my partner, but I'm happy to share."

—Metis Black, founder of Tantus, Inc.

## CYBERSKIN

If a real penis experience is what you're trying to approximate, cyberskin is the most lifelike material on the market. It's a mixture of plastic and silicone, and it's usually super soft but also super difficult to keep clean. It's porous, like jelly rubber, and if it comes into contact with another toy, or oil or silicone lube, it will transform itself anew, and odds are that's not a good thing. Generally cyberskin, realskin, or Ultraskin (same thing, different companies) toys are so porous that using the wrong product, like a silicone lube, on the toy will change its shape, texture, and mold. Similar to jelly rubber, toys made with cyberskin may contain phthalates, but not all of them do. If you want a real-deal toy without phthalates, Topco Sales's CyberSkin toys have been tested by Greenpeace and declared phthalate- and PVC plastic–free.[8]

Now for the even bigger downside. Unlike a real penis, cyberskin doesn't just scrub clean with soap and warm water. After you wash and pat dry your cyberskin toy, you'll need to apply a light layer of cornstarch—c-o-r-n-s-t-a-r-c-h, not talcum powder—to prevent the toy from getting sticky. For further cleaning instructions, check out "Coming Clean (With Your Toys)" at the end of this chapter.

As an educated consumer, you have a right to ask questions about the composition of materials in your toys. To be extra safe, use a condom with all of the "skin" types of toys. On the bright side, it might even make the toy feel more real.

## ACRYLIC

Acrylic toys are hard and smooth, and, like hard plastic, they're great for insertion if you're looking for something that really hits the spot. Unlike hard plastic, acrylic toys don't crack or shatter. Plus, they're super lightweight, so they're easy to maneuver and won't tire out your wrists. And they're phthalate-free. My favorite G-spot toy is an acrylic S-shaped wand. It not only is the perfect curve to hit the spot, but it is so light and easy to hold that I could play with it for hours.

## STAINLESS STEEL

Stainless steel toys are not just hard, cold, and heavy, they are a totally hip way to exercise your PC muscle. You can put them in the fridge or a bowl of warm water to change their temperature. They're easy to clean, but don't use abrasives to clean them because that will dull the look of your toy. Njoy makes superb-quality stainless steel toys. From the Pure Wand (which curves like the letter C, with a large ball on one end and a small ball on the other) to the

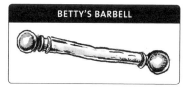

BETTY'S BARBELL

Fun Wand (which has a tail with three graduated balls), stainless steel toys not only are boilable and dishwasher-safe, they are heavier than any other sex toys on the market (the Pure Wand weighs twenty-four ounces and the Fun Wand weighs eleven). Njoy also makes three different-size butt plugs, with different-size heads, but all three have the same unique flared base that fits nicely between each of your butt cheeks.

## GLASS

Glass is also hard, and toys made from glass can be aesthetically spectacular, as both dildos and butt plugs. Companies like Phallix, Xhale Glass, and XXX Glass are into the craftsmanship, quality, and design of their toys. And

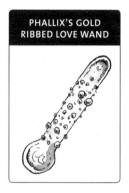

**PHALLIX'S GOLD RIBBED LOVE WAND**

since glass is easily bendable, there are lots of interesting shapes and styles available for your personal enjoyment. You'll find Pyrex glass toys that have hearts blown into their shafts, others that are etched in twenty-four-carat gold, and others that have unique twists, curves, and handles. Quality glass toys, especially Pyrex, are never hollow on the inside, and you don't want to play with a toy that feels hollow, both because that means it's probably cheaply made

and because a hollow toy can break way easier than a solid glass one. Pyrex is, great because it can be boiled, and you can heat it up in water or cool it off in your refrigerator (not freezer) for a quick change in temperature.

> *"I like using glass toys instead of rubber dildos because they don't have a lot of give to them, so they don't flop around everywhere. They don't break and they never wear out, so you can keep them forever. My favorite would be Xhale's Heartbreaker because I like the thickness, and I love the pink hearts!"*
>
> *—Lux Kassidy, age twenty-one*

## STONE

Stone is a material that has been around for ages, but it's only recently found its way back to the sex industry. It's hard, and you can heat it up or cool it down for further titillation. From marble to jade to jasper, a hard rock can substitute for a hard cock any time you want it to.

> "I have a rock—it's called the Massage Stone—that I bought at a spa store. And although they never mention its 'other uses,' it's a phallic-shaped massage stone that's smooth and temperature-cool, and it feels really neat. Mine is made out of travertine and it's my favorite penetrative dildo!"
>
> —Regina, age thirty-five

 **EXTRA! EXTRA!**

Yes, there's a lot to think about when buying sex toys, but the more thought out your prepurchase decision-making is, the more likely you'll be to find the right sex toy for your "right now" needs.

## COLOR

The material that goes inside you might be determined by how many bucks you have to blow, or it might depend on the visual variables of color and style. What should be most important is the quality of the material you'll put in your body, but when I worked as a sex educator at the toy shop Babeland, I saw how color could affect a purchase. Sure, it's a part of the visual process of arousal, but with three exceptions it shouldn't be the most important thing about the toy. Those three exceptions are: (1) When it comes to toys for the bum, a darker color is a better bet than a lighter one. (Darker colors can help alleviate anxiety, especially if you're squeamish about poop.) (2) You're planning on keeping it on the coffee table, and want your toy to match the decor of the room. (3) You only wear one color and everything you own is that color.

If those three reasons don't apply to you, then odds are that when you're masturbating you're not going to care about the color. Besides, what's most important is how it feels in you, or on you.

## CURVY, STRAIGHT, OR BUMPY

Some toys are pinstripe straight, while others are wavy or curved at the tip. Lots of women like curved toys because they're designed to hit the top wall of the vagina and hook around the pubic bone so that they make direct contact with the G-spot. Other women prefer straight toys, whether it's because they feel more comfortable thrusting with them during masturbation, or because the toys themselves can stimulate more surface area than some of their curved counterparts.

Whether you play with curved or straight toys, there may be some other spots you want to check out. Mainly I'd suggest the anterior fornix erogenous (AFE) zone, but you might also want to take a poke at the cervix. The AFE zone, also known as the A-spot, is found closer to the cervix, on the top wall of your vagina (same wall as the G-spot). It's a larger, less defined area than the G-spot, and gentle, lighter strokes work best in this zone (the G-spot requires a firmer stroke). As for the cervix, recent exploration by sex researcher, nurse, and author Beverly Whipple has shown that the cervix has nerve pathways that can produce an orgasmic response.[9] Cervical stimulation won't be every lady's cup of tea, but if it's something you haven't thought about before, it couldn't hurt to sip and see.

Bumpy is most often seen in your garden-variety butt toys, like anal beads or butt plugs. Sometimes bumpy means that the balls gradually build up, especially as you get nearer to the tail of the toy. Bumps are nice when you're having an orgasm, because your muscles can contract around each bead and leave you with a sensational orgasmic experience. You might also enjoy Smartballs, or other spherical objects, while you masturbate. Ultimately any toy can work for you, depending on how you work with it. The great news is that you're not limited to just one tool for your box!

## THICKER OR THINNER

Again, this is a personal preference depending on how stuffed you like to feel. Don't go with anything too thin, unless you seriously can't get anything even a little bit thick inside yourself. Too thin, over time, will start to feel like nothing at all.

 According to Rachel Venning, cofounder of the sex shop(s) Babeland, 65 percent of Babeland's customers (online or in person) are women.[10]

## VIBRATING OR STATIC

If I were going to choose only one toy to fulfill my masturbatory fantasies, I'd definitely go with something that vibrates. It doesn't mean I have to turn it on, but I'd rather have the choice. Of course, you can always add a vibrator to your sex play, whether or not it's attached to the dildo or butt plug you've selected. Nowadays many toys are multifaceted, so you can own as many or as few as you want and still cover all your bases when it comes to the bells and whistles you may want to add to your masturbation repertoire.

> "If I had a vibrating saddle with a dildo attached, now that would be my favorite masturbation toy!"
>
> —Mink, age thirty-six

## A PHTHALATES-FREE GUIDE TO THE "OTHER" SEX TOYS

### DILDOS

**Betty's Barbell:** This heavy (nearly one-pound) stainless steel rod is not only a really nice dildo, it's also a fantastic Kegel exerciser, and it's designed by the grandmother of female masturbation (Ms. Betty Dodson).

**Chinese Jade (the Massage Stone):** Chinese jade is said to be connected with the heart chakra, so give yourself a heart-on with this hard, solid dildo. You can heat it up or chill it down; just be careful not to drop it, because it can break.

**Clear Crystal Wand:** Acrylic, light, and perfectly designed (like an S) to hold on to while you sexplore your G-spot. I must admit that I have a special place in my heart for this one. I wouldn't have had my first G-spot orgasm without it!

**Dolphin Stub, S, M, XL (Funfactory):** This royal-blue dolphin dildo looks like one of those aquarium performers, but (depending on the size) it's got curve. The medium size is arched for maximum spottage, and you can use this silicone toy in either opening because of its flared base.

**Doppeltes Lottchen (Funfactory):** Forget trying to pronounce this one. Instead, focus on the fact that it's a really cute double dildo, meaning you can use on either end, or both ends, inside yourself during masturbation. Pure silicone, it comes in yellow and blue.

**Gold Twist with Handle (Xhale):** This interesting glass dildo is fumed with twenty-four-carat gold and is double-sided for two totally different feels. One side has a more phallic-shaped, traditional head, while the other is twisted and a tad bit pointy. It's ten and a half inches of braided beauty.

**Feeldoe (Erogenics):** Composed of three parts, the pony (the part that goes inside you), the saddle (what you sit on), and the horse (the shaft), the Feeldoe is a uniquely angled silicone dildo that's easy to use. Created by a woman inventor, and distributed by Tantus, Inc., it comes in three sizes—original, slim, and stout. Vibration optional.

**Leo (Vixen Creations):** One of Vixen's best-selling dildos, this realistic (but not too realistic) long silicone dick averages seven inches in length and comes in silver glitter. How fun is that?

**LoneStar (Vixen Creations):** If real is your deal, you've met your match. Made out of Vixen's exclusive VixSkin (which is 100 percent silicone), this chubby dick is average in length but thick in width. And if you order it from Vixen, it's got a lifetime warranty.

**Love Wand (Phallix):** These 100 percent handblown objets d'art are totally worth their weight in gold (some of them even have gold etching). The glass is "doctor-approved" Pyrex, and the colors are etched on the inside so they won't fade away—even if your love for the toy does. Also makes a great conversation piece.

**Lumina Wand:** Molly Ringwald isn't the only one who's pretty in pink. This coolly designed hard acrylic wand is curved to hit the G-spot. Plus, it's super lightweight.

**Pure Wand (njoy):** If you already know that you love stainless steel, or even if you're just curious about it, this is a must-have toy for you. Weighing in at one and a half pounds, and made of twenty-four ounces of the finest medical-grade stainless steel, this curved toy is a big hit among the ladies (and the dudes). With a larger and smaller ball on either end, this toy will help you hit the G-spot. All njoy products are hand-tested (not each specific toy, just each shape and style) to ensure that they get the job done.

**Revolution (Tantus):** Part of the Tantus Dual Density 02 line, Revolution has a Pure Skin outer layer, and a super-firm inner "muscle core." Made of a silicone that doesn't require the care of cyberskin (but feels like it would), this is a great toy for any real-deal enthusiast. Comes in three fun colors—light purple, light blue, and light pink—for the girlie-girl in all of us.

### BUTT STUFF

**Aneros (Aneros):** Once thought of as a maker of boy toys, Aneros has come a long way, baby. Designed by scientists, their newest anal product, the Peridise, is not just for boys anymore. Guys have been going ga-ga over Aneros for quite some time, and now it's time for the ladies to check out an anal PC toy that's designed to create involuntary peristaltic contractions that will make your bum sing.

**Buddy (Vixen Creations):** Vixen's most popular (and silicone) butt plug, Buddy is a stay-put, curved plug that starts smaller and ends wider (but not too wide).

**Corona (Good Vibrations):** This high-quality borosilicate cobalt-blue glass plug is not only easy on the eyes, it's easy on the ass as well. It's got two bulbs for different sensations, and an indent at the bottom that helps it stay in place.

**Flexi Felix (Funfactory):** A seriously cute set of anal beads that looks like a caterpillar (I hope that doesn't sound unsexy, but it's true, in a good way), Flexi Felix will make you smile. Not only is this toy made of silicone, but since all the balls and the string are coated in it, these beads are way more sanitary than your traditional anal beads.

**Infinity (Tantus):** Available in two sizes, the silicone Infinity might be larger than your traditional beginner plug, but it will stop you from getting bored so quickly. Has a great stay-put base to boot!

**Fun Wand (njoy):** Another stainless steel great, the Fun Wand is curved like the letter S and has three smooth, graduated teardrop-shaped balls on one end (the largest being one inch thick), and one larger one-inch head-ball at the tip of the other end. Weighing a little under a pound, this Fun Wand is sleeker and slimmer than its Pure Wand sibling, but both are functionally and sensationally fantastic—whichever end you choose to use.

**Little Flirt (Tantus):** A very, very beginner butt plug, it's literally no bigger than the size of your pinky finger—even if it's a tad bit thicker than that. Great for a first-timer, but you might get bored with this teeny-weeny plug after a while.

**Pure Plug (njoy):** These stainless steel butt plugs have a larger head and smaller stem, and can seriously sit out on your night table because they're so damn stylish. Each is finished off with a little handle, one that you can use to carry the toy, but that also lies between your butt cheeks when it's inside you. It's heavy, too, which doesn't allow you to forget you've got something back there.

**Ripple Plug (Tantus):** Tantus makes some of the best butt plugs, and this is no exception. Sort of like anal beads (only with no string and a flared base), the Ripple features four bumps and comes in two sizes.

**Silicone Anal Beads (Tantus):** Not as cute as Flexi Felix, but if "not as cute" is the way you'd rather go up the butt, then these fantastic and functional silicone anal beads are your best bet. Looks more like a really long butt plug than your traditional beads.

**Tristan 1 (Vixen):** This silicone butt plug was designed to stay in place by the ultimate queen of anal sex, Tristan Taormino. Not to be confused with the bigger, badder, and vibrating-if-you-want-it Tristan 2 (which is another option), the Tristan 1 is great if you want something with a little bit of meat on its bones.

### ADDITIONAL ACCOUTREMENTS

**Clover Clamps:** For fans of some serious nipple clamping, these clamps start out firm, and the more you pull on them, the tighter they become. Attached together by a leather loop or metal chain and originally from Japan, these stay in place better than most other nipple clamps.

**Feathers:** Whether it's a decadent ostrich feather wrapped on a long, elegant crop or a feather boa you got at one of those fashion accessory stores, adding additional, noninvasive stimulants is a sure way to pump up your volume.

**Smartballs (Funfactory):** A safer and larger version of Ben Wa balls, Smartballs are attached by a silicone-coated cord so that they don't float independently inside your vagina. There's a free-floating weight inside each ball, for added massage, and a tamponlike cord at the end for easy outage. Add vibration to the outside of one of the balls, sit back, and let them send you into a tizzy.

**Tweezer Nipple Clamps:** You could probably pluck your eyebrows with these clamps, but you shouldn't. Tweezer clamps come with rubber tips (pull out the Krazy Glue) to protect you from the horrible pain of, well, not having rubber tips. They're adjustable, small and harmless looking.

**Snakebite Kit:** Most people take snakebite kits camping just in case they get bitten by a snake, but you can use the powerful, not painful suction cups (there happen to be three of them) on your nipples, clit, or various other body parts. If you buy the entire kit and aren't planning to see a snake anytime soon, you can throw away the rest of the package, but make sure to keep the large and small suction cups for your personal delight.

**Vibrating Nipple Clamps:** These don't grip like the nonvibrating kind, which means you still might be able to feel the circulation in your chest when in use. They are bulky and take watch batteries, but they will surely drive attention to wherever you place them.

 **LIQUID LOVE**

If you're reading this section thinking you don't need to use lube because you're always either drizzling or drenched, think again. Even if you have more condensation than the city of Seattle, you still need to be prepared because what once was wet won't necessarily stay that way. Women on birth control, on antidepressants, and even at different stages in their menstrual cycle (or going through menopause) will, at one time or another, discover that they've lost that lubricated feeling. Because vaginal lubrication is not always a given, and because some women never lubricate enough to enjoy sex without the additional slippery stuff, lube is a must-have on every sex list. Especially when you use sex toys or play with your butt, you'll want—or need—to lube it up.

Now, before you run out to your local pharmacy to pick up drugstore lube, remember the good news. You come equipped with your own natural lubricant: spit—that substance more technically known as saliva. The bad news is that, thanks to some of the more disgusting porn out there, lots of women are turned off by the idea of using their own saliva to fine-tune their knobs. But spit is not gross, and you don't actually have to hock a loogie to get good mileage from your own salivary juices. Instead, moisten up your mouth, then take your hand and transfer the juice from one palette to the other.

The great thing about spit is that it's natural. The bad thing is that it lasts about as long as the flavor in a stick of Juicy Fruit gum, which means you'll need to keep manufacturing more than you'd need if you just opted for artificial lubrication. Still, if nothing feels better than the real thing, it's good to know you can make your own lube anytime you need it.

You've probably heard of either K-Y Jelly or Astroglide. Both water-based lubes have managed to saturate the personal-lubricant market and can be found at any local or chain drugstore. But just because they're more readily available doesn't make them better. While other popular water-based lubes are not as easy to find in a terrestrial pharmacy, they're well worth the search online.

There are two types of lubes that are great for any type of sex. Those are water-based and silicone. Water-based lubes come in two varieties: those that have glycerin and those that don't. Glycerin is a sugar, but not the kind of sugar you'd want to put in coffee. This explains why a lot of glycerin-based lubes have a slightly sweet taste. Most women use glycerin-based lubes without fear, but women who are prone to yeast infections may want to find a lube without it. "Glycerin-free" products use glycol or vegetable glycerin (both are a little different from plain glycerin). Water-based lubes with glycerin will stay slicker for longer than water-based lubes without. But the trick to reusing your water-based lube (once it's on your skin or the toy) is to rewet the lube. Either use spit or keep a cup of water by your place of masturbation. Both can be applied to revive your lube after it leaves you high and dry.

If slick is the word, then silicone lubes are what you need to know about. Nothing about them is natural, but they last so long it's hard to care. Because they don't naturally wash out of your system like water-based lubes, some women worry about using silicone lubes in their vagina, and on the sheets (yes, they can stain). Anally, silicone lubes will wash out with your regular bowel movements, so you don't have to worry about a thing. Vaginally, however, silicone lube is going to stay in your system longer. It will eventually wash out; that doesn't necessarily mean it's going to bother you, but it's something to be aware of.

Silicone lubes are also nice for massage, but they're bad to use with your silicone and cyberskin toys. Picture, if you can, how in *The Wizard of Oz*, water literally melts the Wicked Witch of the West. That's basically what will happen to your silicone or cyberskin toys if you throw silicone lube on them. It may not happen instantly, but over time the liquid silicone bonds with solid silicone or cyberskin toys and basically transforms the toy into an unusual and unusable version of its once-happy self. That means it's best to stick with a water-based lube if you've got a toy that you want to love you long time.

 According to Durex's *Global Sex Survey 2005*, the top three sexual enhancers around the world are pornography (41 percent), massage oils (31 percent), and lubricants (30 percent).[11]

When I masturbated on video for Betty Dodson, she asked me to use an oil-based lube while I played with myself. At first I wasn't so sure if I should. Having worked as a sex educator at the world-famous Babeland, I had been trained to never promote the use of oil-based lubes (especially since they're not condom-compatible). But she insisted, and how could I say no to the grandmother of masturbation? I thoroughly enjoyed my experience and had a great time, and yet outside of that experience, I haven't touched an oil-based lube. Oil is unquestionably not good for condoms, so it's not a lube that will come in handy if you are using them for safer sex. And, like silicone, it takes a longer time to wash out of your body. So, while I don't recommend it for partnered sex, if it works for Betty Dodson for masturbation, it might work for you, too.

No matter what lube you do decide to use, here's something you need to know: Never buy lubes with nonoxynol-9. Nonoxynol-9 is actually a cleaning agent that can irritate the delicate lining of your vaginal wall, and increase your chances of infection. Plus it tastes gross, can cause rashes, and has a numbing effect. It's definitely being phased out of most lubricants, but still, if you find condoms or a lube that claim to have spermicide, pass them on by. Also, never use lubes or gels that describe themselves as "numbing." Numbing agents don't do anything but make you lose feeling, and if you can't feel what you're doing down there, why would you even bother doing it?

> *"In general I have to use lube that doesn't have glycerin in it because my pussy is very sensitive and I get yeast infections if I sneeze at it wrong. I used to swear by Slippery Stuff, but haven't been using it much lately. These days, depending on what consistency I want, I like Maximus (thicker for anal, though it tastes awful), Sliquid (which has a similar consistency to natural lubricant), and I've also developed a taste for Eros, especially for partnered sex."*
>
> —Audacia Ray, age twenty-seven

**BECAUSE YOU'VE GOT OPTIONS: A GIRLS' GUIDE TO LUBE**

### WATER WORKS: THE KIND WITH SUGAR AND WITHOUT

**Astroglide:** Designed by rocket scientists to feel like the real thing, Astroglide's tagline is, "Second only to nature." Yet, unlike nature, it's thin and slick, and a tad bit stringy, with a slightly sweet taste and a mellow, yet artificial, scent. Its original formula does contain parabens (a preservative that can cause skin irritation and burning, especially if you're hypersensitive to chemicals) and glycerin.

**Durex Play More:** Available at your neighborhood drugstore, this glycerin-free lube doesn't have much of a taste or smell, and it will last long enough for a playdate with yourself. Made from the same company that brings you quality condoms, this is a quality, readily available, funtastic lube.

**Emerita Natural Lube:** Allantoin, a botanical extract, helps promote healthy skin and limit irritation while vitamin E moisturizes in this glycerin-based lube. Created by a woman-owned, woman-operated company, it's got no taste and a slick feel.

**Good Clean Love Almost Naked:** Good Clean Love cares about quality. Made with 100 percent natural ingredients, Almost Naked has no petrochemicals, no parabens, no taste, and a light lemon-vanilla scent, and it's 100 percent vegan. This lube contains vegetable glycerin, a fantastic alternative for the health-conscious woman. Because it's so natural, you will have to relubricate often.

**Hydra Smooth:** *Creamy* comes to mind with this glycerin-free lube. It has a bit of a bittersweet taste, but after an initial dab, it's really not so bad. And it is nice and well, smooth.

**Liquid Silk:** For a lot of women, this name says it all. Another creamy lube without glycerin, Liquid Silk doesn't get sticky and doesn't really smell, but it does taste bitter, really bitter. And even though it's vegan, it does contain parabens.

**Maximus:** Thick and long-lasting, this is a popular lube among the ladies, especially for ass play. It's glycerin-free and clear, but it does have parabens and, like its sister lube, Liquid Silk, it has a strong, bitter taste.

**O'My Natural:** This nice, long-lasting, natural lube contains hemp (without THC), which is supposed to discourage the growth of unwanted yeast and bacteria. It has a little bit of a smell and taste, but it's such an impressive lube, it's easy to ignore them. The first ingredient is glacier water, and instead of regular glycerin, it contains vegetable glycerin.

**Probe Silky Light:** Sweet-tasting and vegan, this stringy lube lists grapefruit seed as one of its only four ingredients. It dries out quickly, though.

**Slippery Stuff Gel:** Originally designed to help divers get into and out of their wetsuits, this lube is one of the best bangs for your buck. It will stay put, but it does dry out quicker than some other lubes, and it's a bit stringy, with a slight taste and odor.

**Sliquid Sassy:** Great packaging, paraben- and glycerin-free, super-thick, and a little foamy, the newest of the Sliquid line will not let you down. With no taste and no smell, it lasts longer than a lot of other water-based lubes.

### WATER-BASED LUBES: TASTE TREATS

**Emerita OH Warming Lube:** There's a faint cinnamon smell to this one, and it warms up on your skin without feeling like you've just doused Ben-Gay on your clit. The ingredients include glycerin, cinnamon bark, and honey, and it has a slightly funny taste. But it's slippery and long lasting.

**ID Juicy Lubes:** I tasted three gel flavors: Big Banana, Luscious Watermelon, and Strawberry Kiwi. While each lube smelled like its name, they all sort of tasted the same—sweet. These flavored lubes contain glycerin and get stringy and sticky over time.

**O'My Strawberry Cheesecake:** The O'My flavored lubes really do taste good. It's like licking the wallpaper in Willy Wonka's chocolate factory: The Strawberry Cheesecake tastes like strawberry cheesecake. Plus, it's sugar-free and contains only vegetable glycerin.

**Sliquid Swirl:** The Blue Raspberry is undoubtedly the best-tasting lube I've ever sampled, because it not only tastes yummy, but also smells delicious. Glycerin-free and sweetened with aspartame, it's easy to use and easy to clean up. Available in other flavors as well, like Green Apple Tart and Cherry Vanilla, both of which also taste good.

### SILICONE-BASED: GREAT FOR MASSAGE, SEX, AND SHAVING!
**Eros (Pjur) Bodyglide:** This German-designed lube is not only the perfect lube, it's also the most popular silicone lube on the market. Smooth, long-lasting, tasteless, and great for massage, it might even outlast the Energizer bunny.

**ID Millennium:** This lube is typically less expensive than some of its contemporaries, but it lacks the consistency of other silicone lubes. Super-thin and a bit drippy, it may cost less, but you're going to use more each time. Still, it has no bad taste or smell.

**Pink:** Although it's risky to put a super-slick lube in a handblown Italian glass bottle, there is something elegant and discreet about Pink. Made with the highest-quality silicone available (dimethicone), vitamin E, and aloe vera, it lotions while it lubes. And the bottle is just so darn pretty.

**Sliquid Silk:** Made with only 12 percent silicone, this mutt of a lube is super slippery, but does have a slightly bitter taste. It's a great combination of water-based and silicone lubes, and it's so delightfully creamy and, again, long-lasting!

**Wet Platinum:** This extra-concentrated silicone lube is also less expensive than certain other brands, but it has a thin, oily consistency and a bad chemical taste.

 **TIP** Want to add a little extra visualization when administering your lubricated love? Wear latex or polyurethane gloves, especially black latex, and notice what it feels like to touch yourself with a barrier.

 ## COMING CLEAN (WITH YOUR TOYS)

Keeping most toys clean is as simple as washing them with soap and warm water and then storing them in a safe, dry place. You should clean your toys both before and after you use them. You don't need to use "adult" toy cleaners because they're basically soap and water. However, with certain materials you can take added measures to ensure that your toy is the king or queen of clean. You can boil Pyrex, silicone, or stainless steel dildos or butt toys (if they come with a separate vibrator, you'll need to take that out first) for two to three minutes, or place silicone and Pyrex in the top rack of your dishwasher (the steam of the dishwasher is great for cleaning silicone toys, and for removing any traces of hepatitis B). Since Pyrex, stainless steel, and silicone are nonporous to begin with, when you're not sharing them, it's easiest to just wash them the way you would hard plastic, acrylic, or jelly rubber, and that's with soap and warm water.

Cyberskin toys do require extra tender loving care and, again, should not be used with silicone lube. After each use, you need to clean your real-skin toy and then let it dry completely, both inside and out, before coating it with a light sprinkling of cornstarch. (Do not use talcum powder, even if your toy comes with it. Throw it out. That stuff has been linked to cervical cancer and should never go inside your vagina.) Then wrap it up, in something like a silky scarf, and put it down to rest. You'll need to repeat this lengthy process after each use of your cyberskin toys (and others like them) because they're extremely porous. You can always use a condom over any sex toy for a lightning-quick clean each and every time.

 ## FOR THE LOVE OF TOYS

Shopping for sex toys can be part of foreplay when it comes to solo sex. It can fill your mind with racy thoughts and juicy ideas. Even if it doesn't work out in the long run, it's nice to change things up. Anybody can use a sex toy, regardless of whether you consider yourself a sinner, saint, slut, or virgin—sex toys don't discriminate. Masturbate with your sex toys and share them with your partner. Love them and they will, in turn, love you back (but not in that human companion sort of way). In a world where we could all use a little more love, who can argue with that?

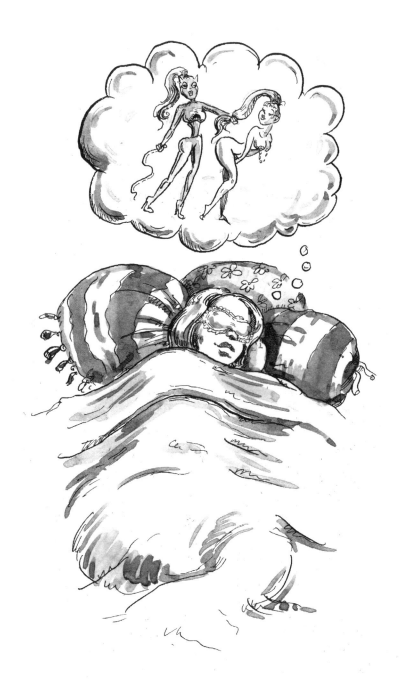

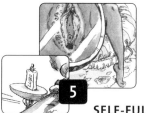

## 5

## SELF-FULFILLING FANTASIES:
### *Fuel for Desire*

IF YOU THINK IT IN YOUR HEAD, and use it in bed, but it's not tangible, available, or even realistic, it's called a sexual fantasy. Sexual fantasy can be a thought, an image, or a detailed and descriptive story that weaves its way through your mind and works to heighten your arousal. Good sexual fantasy is imagery that we create to stimulate and empower ourselves. Good sexual fantasy teaches us to rely on our creativity, imagination, and experiences to generate our own series of smutty and scrumptious thoughts.

When you fantasize, it's all about you. Nobody needs to know what you're thinking, who you're doing, or why you want what you want. Fantasy is a completely natural way to creatively envision your life outside of the confines of what it already is and isn't. Even if you're one of those women who fantasizes only on the third Friday of every fourth month, know that whenever you do fantasize, you're adding a whole other dimension to your fooling around, and you're allowing the most powerful sex organ, your brain, to play a significant role in your arousal and orgasm.

Fantasy is excellent fodder for masturbation. It's a way to play with your imagination, test your boundaries, and think up dirty, delicious, and deviant things you may never want to try outside of your mind. Imagine you are the most famous webcam girl and you're putting on a masturbation show for millions of viewers. Or think about your favorite fairytale and add lots of solo sex to your story of being kept in a tower. Pretend you've been captured, and that your captors are forcing you to masturbate for them, or think about your first kiss and let that lead you to orgasm. Regardless of why or what you choose to invent, or live out, if you're okay going there in your head, then everything else will be okay, too.

You can also act out your fantasies during sex with a partner. You can role-play with your partner and bring your sex life to another dimension. For instance, if you've ever dreamed of being a rock star, your guy can be a lucky groupie who gets to fuck you backstage after a big concert. Or if you've wanted to be a dominatrix, your girlfriend can be your submissive, and you can tie her up to the bed or a chair and tickle-torture her with feathers. Maybe you're into pretending you're from another universe and this is your first day on the planet, and you've knocked on your lover's door looking for some human affection. Or you and your partner can meet at a bar and pretend to be strangers and then sneak into a bathroom, or back alley, to get it on. Whatever your fantasy, when you feel safe and protected you can let your imagination run wild. If you don't feel comfortable fantasizing with your partner, don't sweat it. It's honestly easier to let yourself go (into another time, place, and person) when you're doing it for yourself, by yourself.

##  FUEL FOR YOUR BRAIN

You don't have to think up every one of your fantasies to fuel your own masturbation. Sure, some fantasies are born of personal experience, but plenty of women collect stories and turn-on titillation from books of erotica, adult videos, or steamy sex scenes pulled directly from this summer's biggest box office smash. You can find sexy stories in newsstand magazines like *Penthouse, Playboy,* or *Playgirl,* or on cable channels like Cinemax—especially "after dark." Other women turn to chick lit or romance novels to find a large and diverse selection of fantasy material. That's right: All you have to do is put yourself in someone else's shoes, or watch as someone else's steamy story unfolds in your mind, and you will have found yourself a new adventure of your own. Then you can test out your fantasies while you masturbate. Thinking about sex is a very important part of doing it. Incorporating your brain with your hands can lead to mind-expanding orgasms.

 According to the Romance Writers of America, 5,994 romance titles were released in 2005, and romance fiction generated $1.4 billion in sales that same year.

Not all sexual fantasy is candy and roses, and not everyone fantasizes about happy, beautiful things. Some fantasies are not politically correct. Even if you can't fathom or wish for something in real time, you can still wank off to it in your alone time. There's nothing wrong with imagining yourself being forced to have sex (yes, that's rape with a lowercase "r"— and it can happen in your head without any judgment) or getting gang-banged by the entire college football team. Remember, because it's fantasy, it's different from what you'd experience in real life. In fact, you may not actually wish for the things you fantasize about to come true in real life, which is both freeing and perplexing. But reality bites sometimes, while fantasy doesn't even leave a mark. Of course, there is such a thing as bad sexual fantasy, which is imagery that you use to make yourself feel guilty or ashamed, or that serves as a reminder of a past experience that you may feel you deserved. Nobody deserves to torture him- or herself with evil fantasies, unless the truth is that you get off on this type of self-abuse and don't actually find your negative thoughts unhealthy in your regular world. If that's not the case for you, though, try to focus on where you're at when you feel yourself going to a bad headspace. Think about how or what you're feeling, or about having an orgasm, to condition yourself to eradicate any bad thoughts or poor self-image.

## NANCY FRIDAY: EXPOSING OUR SEXUAL IMAGINATIONS

Nancy Friday is a feminist writer, researcher, and journalist who, during the late 1960s and early 1970s, earned her spot in the new women's movement by seeking out ways to explore female, and later male, sexuality and relationships. In June 1973, she published her groundbreaking book, *My Secret Garden*. Prior to that, no one had written about women's fantasies. There were no references on the subject in the New York Public Library, there was no Internet to surf, and there was no place to go to find out what women were thinking when they had sex. Friday revealed the detailed, erotic, and kinky types of sexual imagery that women got off to, including adultery, exhibitionism, group sex, lesbianism (for lots of women who identified as straight), sex with in-laws or other family members, sex with someone dead, famous, or imagined, nonconsensual sex, threesomes, dominance, and submission. She shed light on the fact that there isn't one flavor all women like, and that for some women vanilla is a total drip. Friday showed the world that women are turned on by lots of different switches, and that there isn't one lever that controls the sexual fantasies for all womankind.

On the darker side, she discussed some of the less politically correct or pretty aspects of fantasy. Her book received a lot of praise, but also a fair share of criticism and disgust. The very same month *My Secret Garden* was published, *Cosmo* ran a cover story by Dr. Allan Fromme, a well-known clinical psychologist who went so far as to state that women don't have sexual fantasies because they don't enjoy sex! The success of Friday's first book led to the completion of two more, and this trilogy of books on female sex fantasies not only was enough to prove this particular doctor wrong, but was proof positive that women weren't simply lying on their backs when it came to sexual pleasure.

Wherever you get your fantasy fuel from, make sure to keep your tank full of ideas, stories, and suggestions so that you can add a little extra to your masturbation preparation. A personal favorite of mine comes from the original *Revenge of the Nerds*. There's a scene where nerdy Louis meets Pi Delta Pi's Betty Childs in one of those moon-bounce machines you'd find at a carnival. He's wearing a Darth Vader costume so you can't see his face, and she's dressed in a cheerleader costume (yes, way too unoriginal, but it's still really hot). What I like most about watching her get it on with this geek is that she has no idea who he is, and actually thinks he's her "hunky" boyfriend, Stan. And they have this amazing, beautiful sex and he never even takes his mask off. I like to masturbate when I think of this scene, and I don't necessarily feel the urge to be in it, or change up the action. Since there was no graphic sex in the movie, it allows me to make things happen the way I'd want them to. And that's certainly one way to work on your fantasies. They can include you, or you can just watch as other people fornicate for your personal pleasure. It's all up to you where you let your mind wander.

> "I don't really have any fantasies. I usually focus on getting that warm feeling going between my legs. Sometimes I replay recent sexual episodes that I've had with other partners, but that's the extent of my fantasy life."
>
> —Ilene, age twenty-six

"I swear I used the same Anaïs Nin story from her book Delta of Venus *for at least ten years. I did feel a little weird about it, because it's got this whole pedophilia, and then incest, thing going on, but I tried to just go with it and not deconstruct it too much. For some reason, Faulkner really turns me on, too. Almost any time I read Faulkner— any passage, even those that are not explicit or actually sexual—I get turned on and end up masturbating. Lately I've been getting into more gender-fuck fantasies where I have a dick, and they're always in places like Chaucer's England. I'm usually fucking farmers' wives on utilitarian wooden chairs in old kitchens while the husband sleeps upstairs, pushing up their layers of skirts, wearing boots, and knowing I'll continue walking along the country road in a few hours. Generally, my own fantasies, or text erotica, turn me on more than photos and videos."*

—Kovner, age twenty-eight

 **THINKING SEX**

Fantasies don't have to be overly descriptive in order to work; in fact, they can be one line that triggers an emotional experience in your body. Just thinking about lying on the beach while you watch a nubile, strapping lass play volleyball can take you to another place, or maybe imagining how a lover touches your hand, your face, or other body parts does it for you. While some people come up with fantasies that others might not dream up in a million years, there are lots of core fantasies that the majority of women enjoy. Following are some of the more prevalent themes of sexual imagery.

## WATCHING OR BEING WATCHED

Lots of women masturbate thinking about someone watching them. Some women go so far as to keep the blinds up and the windows open, just for the titillation of thinking someone might happen along and sneak a peek inside. Whether your fantasy is about a group of Trojan warriors stumbling across you masturbating in a meadow, or about just spying on other people getting off while you're sitting, unassuming, on a park bench, exhibitionism and voyeurism are total turn-on material.

> *"My favorite fantasies involve people watching me. Sometimes I'm on a beach blanket and other people watch me touch myself. Other times I'm in my doctor's office and all the people in reception are watching as I entertain them."*
>
> —Thea, age thirty-one

## LESBIAN SEX

Lots of women fantasize about having sex with someone of the same sex, even though not all women actually go out and get it on. For some of us, the fantasy of touching another woman's breasts, pussy, or the soft skin at the top of her inner thighs is enough to get us touching ourselves. Other women may use a same-sex experience they've had before as fodder for fantasy, even if they are no longer sexual with women.

"I used to fool around with women, and now I'm partnered and not that sexually free anymore, so I fantasize about having sex with women, usually random women I see on the subway or something like that. I once saw a sexy woman in the summer with her blouse unbuttoned a little too much, and she wasn't aware of it, or was pretending not to be aware, and she leaned over and her shirt was a little see-through and her breasts were falling out of her bra a little, like spilling over, and she was just so amazingly sexy in that moment. I fantasize about rubbing up against her on the train, or going home with her. When I see something sexy, it just sparks my imagination."

—Christen, age thirty-four

"Typically, I envision a beautiful European woman going at it with some blond American slut. In my mind they've just finished taking a swim in the pool and their long-time friendship creates a sexual tension, so they decide to experiment. Incidentally, they're both so attractive they could be models. Now that I think about it, my scenario sounds like a clichéd scene out of a cheap porn movie. The whole thing is kind of strange, especially since I'm not lesbian, let alone bisexual. Maybe if I were, I could reenact some of the fantasies I have when I masturbate."

—Brittany, age eighteen

## ROLE REVERSAL

In this fantasy, you aren't you, at least not in the way you see yourself regularly. For example, someone who sees herself as shy, introverted, and submissive might fantasize about being dominant, self-assured, and loud when it comes to how she likes to have sex. Or, if you are a dominant, tie-someone-else-up-and-take-control sort of gal, maybe you fantasize about being meek and easily manipulated. This act of reversing your reality self with your fantasy self is an all-time favorite fantasy for a lot of women. You can also reverse yourself in terms of gender. If you are a woman, you might try visualizing yourself as a dude, complete with penis, or maybe you keep your body but experiment with a dildo and harness. If you fantasize about stroking your cock or sticking your prick in someone else's hole, but most of the time you are all about getting something shoved inside of you, you're having another kind of mind-bending, gender-fucking fantasy. These types of fantasies can put you in control, or take away your control, depending on your needs and desires.

"I have standby fantasies. One is that I'm having sex with a woman, either my girlfriend or another random woman, and our clits are hard and erect enough to stimulate each other just by rubbing together. In this third fantasy I'm usually a butch dyke (which I'm not in real life) and I imagine that I'm like the William McNamara character in the Jodie Foster movie Stealing Home and I've gone to visit this girl with the intention of asking her to go out with my best friend. Only she's totally aggressive and she makes the moves on me. We're both wearing underwear from this bygone era, the kind that covers way too much flesh for something that you wear under your other garments. But it's her straightforwardness and these conservative undergarments that really turn me on. Well, and the fact that her mother is just upstairs, unaware of her aggressive, seductive daughter in the living room."

—Shannon, age thirty-three

## STRANGER SEX

Lots of women visualize a particular person when it comes to their fantasies, but many others don't put a face or a name to their fantasy fuck. If masturbating to a body type works for you, then fantasize your perfect partner without a head, or fantasize someone with rotating heads, like the bad guy Man-E-Faces from *He-Man*. And go into detail when you create your sex creature. Does he or she have a thick ass? A toned body? Bulging biceps? You design, you decide.

> "My fantasies generally change a lot during masturbation. I usually begin by imagining that I am meeting someone new and that the chemistry is super strong. We start kissing, touching, and eventually fucking, but the person and place changes with my mood. If I'm lonely and needing affection, then I fantasize that we fall in love, and then the sex is sweet and sensual and he's constantly praising me. If I'm just horny, I like to make it so that I feel totally nasty and dirty, and then I imagine myself in a more taboo situation, something like sex with a stranger or strangers, a husband and wife or another threesome combination. Still, I'll change the scenario instantaneously and continuously if it's not what I need at that moment."
>
> —Misha, age thirty-five

> "My favorite fantasy right now is being strapped to a gurney and rushed into the emergency room. EKG electrodes attached to my chest, oxygen mask covering my nose and mouth, and an IV placed into my arm. As I arrive in the ER, a sexy, super-hot doctor rushes to my side. He begins

> by fondling my clit as he checks my vital signs. Since I am tied down, I cannot move, so my pussy starts dripping with juice as he runs his fingers all over my sweaty body. He pulls down his sexy scrubs to reveal his hard, thick, long, beautiful cock. He gets on top of me on the gurney and voraciously we start fucking, EKG monitoring my every heartbeat. I come and then he sends me back in the ambulance, only to be ravaged by two more sexy paramedic guys. Finally, they drop me off at home with some chocolate chip cookies."
>
> —Lexi Bardot, age twenty-nine

## THREESOMES AND GROUP SEX

Imagining yourself with your two best friends, or at a party where everyone gets a tad too tipsy and proceeds to take off all their clothes and screw on the sofa, on the carpet, and in the master bedroom, is a totally hot fantasy. Sharing your partner with another woman or man is also an easy way to make yourself horny. Of course, if you're one of those jealous types, remember that this is just fantasy and you don't have to ever act it out in reality. But the jealousy you manifest emotionally as you visualize your partner being devoured by a third party may actually lead to more passion in your own self-love, and partnersex, sessions.

> "My favorite fantasy involves three of us, me and two men, and one of those men is sometimes my husband, but not always. I don't actually even participate in the sex; I just watch because I like the idea of two men doing anything and everything together.
>
> —Minna, age thirty-four

"I am walking deep in the woods. It's pitch-black except for a moon pregnant with milky yellow. I am in something really sexy—it changes from a see-through gown to a blood-red corset and panties. I am running and feeling amazing. I lean against big old trees and hump them, play with my yoni, pull at my nipples, laugh, howl, and run some more. I get to a clearing and there is a blazing fire. I look around and sitting toward the cusp of the clearing and forest is the most amazing-looking man, naked, dark-skinned, huge, and he begins ripping on a drum, pounding it so deeply that my entire body vibrates. And then I realize that just beyond the clearing is a cliff and beyond the cliff is the ocean, because I can hear the waves pounding along with the drum. I start to dance, the sexiest temple trance dance I've ever danced. Somehow I've obtained silk scarves and I dance with those and I dance over to the drummer and try to seduce him. He stares me down, like he wants me, like he can taste me, like he wants to devour me. He has a slight vampire vibe and it makes me even hotter. I try to straddle him but he grabs me hard and turns me around, and then there are three other women walking toward us—they are wrapped in some kind of scarves that are pretty much falling off them and they are totally amazing, glowing, tribal, sexy, strong. And before you know it we are all dancing, stripping, pounding our feet into the earth, sweating, and little by little each one of us starts to rub and dance against each other, and then we use rocks and leaves and bark to get each other off, and we are making love with each other and the man keeps on pounding the drum."

—M. B., age thirty-two

## UNTHINKABLE SEX

Fantasies about incest, rape, abduction, bestiality, children, or anything else that's totally taboo—and illegal—in the real world would shock and disgust the most liberal of mothers, and even make Madonna's *Sex* book seem PG. But, it being fantasy, nobody needs to know where your head's at. A mother might fantasize about having sex with her sons to initiate them into adulthood; a high school teacher might fantasize about making the grade with a student. A rape victim might fantasize about raping someone else; another woman might imagine being abducted and forced into sex. We all have a dark side, and we all think disturbing thoughts, and though you might wonder where they come from, they are another aspect to us, and human nature. So even though we can suppress our shadow side, when we're alone, thinking for ourselves, we don't have to.

 The largest published survey on the psychology of sexual fantasies was conducted by psychotherapist Brett Kahr and the British Sexual Fantasy Research Project. Published in 2007, Kahr's research includes the sexual fantasies of nineteen thousand adult U.K. men and women, and his findings show that a large majority of Britons fantasize often. A lot of their fantasies are aggressive in nature, involving some form of harm.

> *"My fantasies usually include a rape scene, where a woman is 'taken' by an older, ugly man, or a young man, and is forced to perform oral sex on him, and then he makes her take it up the ass."*
>
> *—Salka, age thirty-three*

## PAST LOVERS

Lots of women get all verklempt when they think of the one who got away, or the one who took "it" (meaning their virginity) away or taught them how to love, how to fuck, or how to beg for more. Whether you use your past experiences to get off or not, women everywhere use the juicy details of their historic pasts to continue to please themselves in the present.

> "I've been thinking a lot about this guy I was seeing over the summer. We had crazy, passionate, mindless sex—sometimes in inappropriate locations, like my friend's couch while she was in the living room with us, and in the swimming pool at my parents' house. It was very intense, whether we fucked slow or fast, and I like to think about the way he would grab me, bury his face in between my breasts, or bite my earlobe, my shoulder, or the side of my neck. I usually come when I think of him thrusting into me and ejaculating inside of me."
>
> —Lindsay, age twenty-two

> "I often go back to fooling around with my junior high boyfriend in the barn near his house, only in my pretend version we don't just make out. And I was recently very turned on by a spanking fantasy letter in Penthouse. Which is so funny, because I've never gone for that in real life!"
>
> —Jess, age thirty-seven

## KINKY SEX

Fantasies involving rope, bondage, dominance, submission, whips, canes, and paddles are ways to create a power dynamic in your self-sex life. Imagine yourself all tied up and unwilling to do anything but submit to pleasure, or covering up the eyes of a lover while you tease her with your tongue. Or imagine getting disciplined for looking at your partner with a devilish smile, or doing the punishing when your partner speaks without asking permission. Kinky sex adds an extra element of wickedness to your visualization sensations.

> "Recent months have me obsessed with a man I want to peg. I've never considered dominating a man to such an extent before, but this man brings it out in me. I've been fantasizing about nailing his ass—he truly does have the best ass and most beautiful penis I've ever seen. I get off on the fantasy of being able to have power, and at the same time being wanted and knowing that I'd give him pleasure. To me, the ultimate fantasy is being wanted."
>
> —Dusty, age forty-three

> "My favorite fantasy involves a man getting me so worked up and then withholding my pleasure/orgasm until I beg for release. Dirty talk is definitely involved, and sometimes people are watching. I like these control fantasies, but I don't know if I want them to translate into reality. The realm of fantasy is safe and fun, and taboo fantasies can happen in this realm. And I like that . . . a lot."
>
> —Alissa, age twenty-five

## FUCKING YOURSELF FILTHY

Even if you aren't a three-hole type of girl, you might try imagining, at least once, that you want every orifice stuffed up with sex toys, dicks, fingers, and tongues, or any other object that gets you off and gets your mind racing. Again, you don't have to grab two dildos and a ball gag to get this fantasy right; you just need to pretend that you did, and visualize yourself all clogged up and on the verge of coming.

> "My favorite fantasy is where I'm on top of a woman and she's biting and kissing my breasts and I'm rubbing up against her clit with mine and feeling her breasts and a man is penetrating me from behind, holding my ass in his hands while he fucks my pussy."
>
> —Sparks, age twenty-eight

## GETTING PAID FOR SEX

Another hot fantasy involves the exchange of money for services. Whether you fantasize that you're a stripper working the pole, or a prostitute working the streets, it pays off to fantasize about sex work.

> "Sometimes I pretend that I'm the featured dancer at this club in New York and I'm totally untouchable, but everyone wants a piece of me. This one time though, a guy I've seen before approaches me right after I finish my last set. He's dressed to the nines. He's been watching me dance for months, and we've made eye contact before. Tonight he's got something on his mind, and he waves $10,000 under my nose. I grab the money and lead him back to my

➡

*private dressing room and give him the best lap dance ever. Then he rips off my panties and sticks his finger up my cunt. He gets me off, over and over, and when I can't take it anymore, I fuck him. We fuck for hours, until the club is about to close, and then he buttons up his suit, throws another wad of cash on my dressing room table, and leaves, and I don't know if I'll ever see him again."*

—Bunny, age twenty-eight

## NAUGHTY NARRATION

Writing your own erotic narrative, even if it's just in your head, provides you with a healthy dose of sexual sustenance. Maybe this means creating a scenario about an office where the secretary screws her boss, as well as the rest of the high-powered executives. Or it can be a situation between a masseuse and her client, or a vampire and her victim. Whatever story you come up with, enjoy watching the tale unfold in your mind, and feel the effects of the story on your body.

*"The typical fantasies I keep in mind are the schoolgirl/teacher and the hot secretary/boss. Both start with an attraction and innocent flirting, which leads to the teacher/boss catching a glimpse up the schoolgirl/secretary's skirt. From there he masturbates at his desk—when he's alone, but thinking of her, and she always walks in and catches him. When she sees what he's doing she offers to help, and she goes down on him and then sits on him and fucks him, and eventually he bends her over the desk, shirt ripped open and full breasts bouncing. Yep, that's my fantasy."*

—Alli, age twenty-four

**SWEET DREAMS**

John Lennon may have been a dreamer, and he's not the only one, but not every woman devotes time and attention to her imagination. Even if you aren't one of those "free your mind and the rest will follow" types, it's actually emotionally beneficial to give it a try, whenever you have the time to concentrate on your thoughts. You don't have to do it only while masturbating, although that's always a perfect opportunity to give it a go, especially since masturbation is a time when you feel relaxed, zoned out, zoned in, and ready to commit some time to yourself.

 The 1994 *Sex in America* study found that "women who fantasize and use autoerotic materials the most are those who find the greatest number of other sexual experiences appealing."[1]

Wherever and whenever you do it, fantasizing can help you uncover and discover parts of yourself you didn't know existed. You can be someone completely out of your element, or desire something that's so not you (or so you think). Whatever the outcome, fantasy can help you open up to new experiences and expand your awareness of who you are.

Fantasies can also prepare you for something you want to try in your real life. If you continue to fantasize about being tied up and spanked, but the closest you've come is in your mind, then the more you create and explore your story, the more likely the desire is to build up in your loins and prompt you to try it with a willing and trustworthy partner. Until you do, the fantasy and the possibility of turning it into reality will fuel the masturbation fire for sure.

Whatever your reasons for giving yourself permission to let your imagination run wild, let it go. Unhook the leash and see where it takes you. You can learn a whole lot about yourself when you grant yourself the freedom and permission to be whoever it is you want to be.

## ADULT ENTERTAINMENT

Adult entertainment can mean going to a strip, fetish, or sex club, or it can mean renting a porn movie or reading a book or magazine that includes sexy words, sexy acts, or sexy photographs. The purpose of adult entertainment is to bring a tingling sensation to your erogenous zones, mainly the space between your thighs—but every bend and bulge of your bodacious body can, and may, be turned on by dirty words and sexy images. Turn to chapter 9, "Enticement," to find a load of resources designed to appeal to your prurient interests. But for now, let's turn to film.

> *"I don't really have fantasies—meaning things I fantasize about happening to me. Instead I like using porn. It allows me to be a total voyeur."*
>
> —Blythe, age thirty-two

### THE RISE OF DIRTY PICTURES

The briefest of short histories: Before there were dirty movies, there were dirty pictures. Old-time sepia photos and postcards emerged sometime in the late 1800s, and mainstream adult entertainment, in the print form, became universally successful with the creation of *Playboy* in 1953, followed in 1965 by *Penthouse,* and in 1968 by the much dirtier, more descriptive *Screw. Playgirl,* the first newsstand porn magazine for women, came about in 1973 during the feminist movement, as a form of entertainment for sexually liberated women.

The early part of the twentieth century saw the invention of film, and as soon as people were making movies, they were making movies that showed people having sex. These first films, called "stag films," were sepia or black-and-white silent videos that generally had very little plot and a lot of fucking. The heterosexual porn industry as we know it today didn't truly exist until the early 1970s, when two famous films, *Deep Throat* and *Behind the Green Door,* were released in 1972. The difference between those films and today's pornography is that those two films actually had budgets and were produced and directed like most other movies you pay to see at the theater. And hordes of people did see *Deep Throat* in theaters across the nation; it grossed upwards of $100 million before VHS and DVD ever existed and it continues to be one of the highest grossing films to date. Years later, as the VCR became a staple in most households, porn was credited for its success and ubiquity.

Today, thanks to the advent of inexpensive video cameras and the Internet, way more movies are being produced and distributed than ever before, and anybody out there with a camera and a connection can call herself a director. Because there are so many styles and versions of blue movies, a.k.a. porn, in existence (for example, XX-rated movies can't show erect penises, anal sex, penetration, or gynecological shots of vaginas; XXX means hardcore with no restrictions), finding a video that works to fuel your fantasy world may not happen right away. There are lots of porn experts and critics who can help you on your way, but ultimately what you like is not something that anyone else will be able to decide for you.

### WHY WATCH PORN? WHY READ EROTICA?

Even if you can think up every imaginable fantasy, there are still some ideas out there that are beyond your experiences, imagination, or capacities. Therefore erotica, in any form, is a great way to borrow other people's sexual ideas and images. Watching other people's fantasies come to fruition, either in video form or through the turning of pages, can help spark us emotionally, creatively, and sexually. Porn and erotica, photos and text, are great ways to get ourselves going, enjoying our innate desire to watch and/or be watched.

According to the 1994 *Sex in America* survey, 11 percent of women had purchased X-rated movies or videos in the twelve months prior to the publication of the study.[2]

Most of us are voyeurs. Even if we don't "need" to watch, when we get the chance to watch we won't turn it down. Most of us wouldn't mind finding ourselves in a secret sort of cloak-and-dagger position that allows us to watch other people poke and shag. When we tap into the intimate universes of others, we get turned on too. And adult performers provide exactly that: They allow us a window into their intimate moments, where the real orgasms are better than the fake ones, and allow us to explore our own sexuality through watching them display theirs. Written words allow us to envision our own characters while borrowing from the author's real or fictionalized experiences. Like radio, written text allows us to gain admission to the theater of the mind. All positively made erotica is good for our own sex education. Once you discover something that turns you on, you'll feel like you have more options when it comes to getting aroused.

## WOMEN-MADE FANTASIES

Even though more men make erotic movies than women, and most movies are still made for the larger percentage of men who purchase them, there is a nice niche of women writers, directors, and producers who have, or are, making their own mark. When it comes to written erotica, Susie Bright, Alison Tyler, and Rachel Kramer Bussel are three standouts in the field of many women writers who've helped to prove that the pen is a gateway to sexual fantasy. In film, while a majority of the industry ignores the fact that women are visual creatures, there have been, and are, female directors out there who have made, or are making, movies that speak to the growing, empowered female market. Jane Hamilton, who performed under the porn name Veronica Hart, is one such director. Her videos are story oriented, but she directs the sex hard, and raunchy, and includes things like close-ups and cum shots. Sex educator Tristan Taormino has been successful with her line of *Chemistry* videos, and Joanna Angel is both an actress and a director at the forefront of the alt-porn movement. Overseas, Anna Span is a director in Britain whose movies are fun, and whose actors and sex are genuinely hot. Pioneering the couples' market is Femme Productions' Candida Royalle, the woman responsible for creating the "couples-friendly" erotica genre. Her videos are plot driven and do have story-line sex, but there are few cum shots and very little anal. Royalle is continuing to add fresh, young female directors to the mix at Femme Productions, and she recently started producing a second line of videos, *Femme Chocolat*, aimed at a more culturally diverse audience. For a more complete list, check out the resources in chapter 9.

 ## NEVER-ENDING STORIES

Fantasy is a part of reality, and when it comes to our sex lives, if we fantasize we get to explore whole new pathways to our sexuality. So embrace your sexual fantasies, enjoy them, and learn to use them for good things like masturbation, and not for bad things, or in lieu of real life. Always keeping in mind the difference between fantasy and reality is a sure way to keep you out of trouble in the real world, but having fantasies is nothing to be ashamed of, or to feel embarrassed or guilty about. If you find some of your turn-ons bothersome, and you don't want to think about certain things that you can't quite get out of your mind, you can try to distract yourself in the moment by playing music, reading erotica, or focusing on how you feel, as opposed to what you're thinking about to get there. The erotic imagination is a powerful, complex, beautiful, and seductive tool, and only you can control what's been given to you.

There are no limits to your fantasies or your imagination. If you don't see your favorite, or your most reliable, fantasy among the ones presented in this chapter, don't worry. Whatever your fantasy is, it's legit, and you're not the only one who's having such thoughts. Fantasies are healthy, even if they aren't things you'd give yourself permission to act out in your everyday life. Sexual fantasy is great because it allows you to tell your own story, to rewrite parts of your own sexual past and present, and it gives you the visions you need to reclaim yourself as a sexual goddess in the here and now.

We all daydream, fantasize, or snap out of reality sometimes, and fantasies aren't always sexual in nature. They may be about winning the lottery or starring in your own reality TV show. Of course, they could also be about ramming your tongue down Johnny Depp's throat, or wanting a threesome with Posh and Becks. Whatever they are, we all have something we'd love to have happen, even if we're pretty sure it won't.

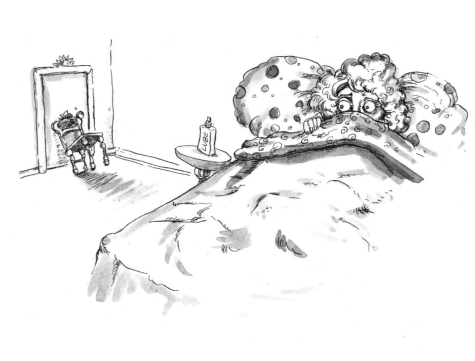

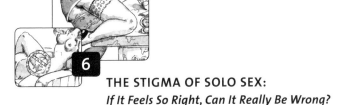

## THE STIGMA OF SOLO SEX:
### *If It Feels So Right, Can It Really Be Wrong?*

IF MASTURBATION FEELS GOOD, can it really be bad? That's the million-dollar question in a society that flaunts its repressive attitudes toward sex. We live in a place where millions of preachers, teachers, parents, and concerned citizens promote a world without touch, at least until marriage, and then and only then in bed with the person you've legally bound yourself to. These "upstanding citizens" have spent years trying to downplay the health and emotional benefits of self-love. But if we think about it, who really has the right to tell us that it's not okay to touch ourselves, that it's not okay to find ways to make ourselves feel good? Telling someone that it's bad to love herself is silly, impractical, and backward.

Still, touchless propagandists rely on social conditioning, which has taught us that good girls don't do nasty things and that masturbation's only for losers who can't get laid. Growing up, we may have gotten slaps on the wrist and eye-rolls of disgust when we loved ourselves without the slightest tinge of guilt or shame. If we're lucky enough to have come from an open family, or perhaps are simply brave or naive, we touch ourselves regardless. We think (and know) that it feels good, and if nobody else knows we're doing it, how bad can we really be? Still, something happens and we fear getting caught, as well as shamed, embarrassed, and punished for loving our own bodies. We associate this fear with the fact that masturbation is talked about as if it were dirty, sleazy, back-alley sex. It takes years, sometimes decades, for women to learn the truth about getting off: The fact is that it's the best way to worship your body, to get to know yourself better—and, with a few small clauses, it's the safest sex you can have.

Back in the day, terms like *hysteria, frigidity,* and *nymphomania* were commonly thrown around to scare women away from sexual activity while reinforcing negative messages about being too sexy. In Victorian times, a woman caught touching herself could be labeled a nymphomaniac and might even be treated with a horrific dose of sulfuric acid dripped directly onto her clit. A woman with hysteria may have been tied down and touched. A masturbator may have had her clit surgically removed.[1] Any sex without a male partner and not for the purpose of procreation was seen as damaging and wasteful to the frail female form.

> *"A new federal report says federally funded sex education programs are telling our children that abortion leads to suicide, that AIDS is transmitted through tears, and that masturbation can result in pregnancy. Do you believe it? Are our tax dollars going to raise a generation of ignorant boobs?"*
>
> —*James Carville, cohost of CNN's* Crossfire[2]

Before the 1870s, when Louis Pasteur showed the world that humans coexist with these things called germs, masturbation was blamed for infections like syphilis and gonorrhea, as well as for infertility and dementia. Masturbation was also linked to cancer, genital shrinkage, acne, blindness, heart disease, and anorexia. And even if masturbation didn't cause nervous disorders or other ailments, its continued practice definitely was thought to aggravate any disease. Women were told that masturbation could lead to an early death and a loss of overall sensitivity. And although we now know that all of the negative hype surrounding the subject is false, we also know that myths linger longer than the scent of a man wearing too much cologne, and the next generation will have to relearn what we already know.

---

**MASTURBATORS BEWARE: 19TH- AND 20TH-CENTURY TECHNIQUES TO PREVENT MASTURBATION IN CHILDREN**

- Prevent sweat buildup (sweat is a possible cause of irritation that might lead to masturbation) with cold showers or swimming.

- Limit the amount of fluids children ingest. Urination draws too much blood—and awareness—to the genitals. Before bed, make them sleepy with medicinal teas.

- Avoid certain foods like artichokes, beans, and peas because they can swell the genitals, as well as spices, rich meats, and venison because of their "aphrodisiacal properties."

- Make sure children get enough exercise so they get tired, but not exercise that allows extra friction to occur. That means children should not climb trees if they must hug their bodies tightly around the trunks. Girls should also avoid horseback riding.

- Marry them off. Marriage is the ultimate guarantee in the prevention of masturbation.

- Tie their hands to the bed rails while they sleep.

- Terrify them with the mere mention, or sight, of knives, scissors, or surgical instruments. Just the threat of cutting their genitals should be enough to scare them into submission.[3]

## HYSTERIA IS NO LAUGHING MATTER

*Hysteria* comes from the Greek word *hystera*, which literally translates to "uterus." When we think of someone who's hysterical, we often think of a person who's so funny that they should be paid to professionally entertain the masses, or someone who's on the brink of a nervous breakdown. But *hystera* means "womb," the place in a woman's body that houses a fetus until birth. And so, aside from being a celebrated place of central importance to life, it has, for centuries, been a supposed central place for irrationality, irritability, and emotional excess. *Hysteria* became an overused diagnosis for any "female" disease, from faintness to irritability to shortness of breath to stress. In fact, in the seventeenth century, fever was the only more commonly diagnosed disease.[4] Hysteria was a medical condition linked to the womb, and it did not have a defined set of indicators, a point driven home when a Victorian physician compiled what he called an "incomplete" list of seventy-five pages of possible symptoms of the disease. Remedies included marriage and pelvic massage, which, in less scientific terms, meant that doctors brought female patients to orgasm.[5] In the late 1800s, the electromechanical vibrator was introduced into medical practices, and from then on masturbation with a vibrator was the reigning champion of hysterical cures. When vibrators became smaller and more readily available, women didn't need to pay doctors to help them relieve their hysteria. They learned to do it on their own, in the privacy of their homes.

 In 1980, the American Psychiatric Association officially changed the diagnosis of hysteria, from "hysterical neurosis, conversion type" to "conversion disorder."[6]

## CAUSE AND EFFECT: MASTURBATION

Masturbation was blamed for lots of people's problems. Here's a list of a few of the ailments once thought to be a result of too much jilling off:

- Acne
- Loss of sight and hearing
- Heart palpitations
- Hysteria
- Insanity
- Lethargy
- Paralysis
- Premature death
- Stunted growth
- Stupidity
- Weight loss

## TAKING THE "SHUN" OUT OF MASTURBATION

Throughout the centuries, it's been quite clear why people have feared masturbation. From hairy palms to premature death to second-rate sex and desperation, there have been a lot of reasons to not do it. But, since nobody's ever died from masturbating, and since masturbators continue to happily procreate, masturbation has carried on, becoming more and more of a mainstream sex habit.

Masturbation, like any sexual activity, is great for your skin and overall health. It improves your circulation, helps build up your immune system, and can lift your mood. And masturbation, unlike other sexual activities, won't make you pregnant or spread disease. It will help boost your self-confidence, will teach you about your favorite erogenous zones, and can help you relax and release any pent-up sexual tension or stress. Regardless of the happy benefits of masturbation, there are still people with concerns about getting off. Here are some of those concerns, broken down for your viewing pleasure.

## MASTURBATION LEADS TO BLINDNESS, HAIRY PALMS, AND DEATH

The fact of the matter is that there are no short- or long-term negative effects of pleasuring yourself. Masturbation does not lead to blindness. You will not grow any, or additional, hair on the palms of your hands. Masturbation will not make you crazy, as in mental-illness crazy, and it will not be the cause of your premature death or any other debilitating diseases. Yes, it can tire out your fingers and/or wrists from time to time, especially during those extended late-night sessions, but it will not stunt your growth or make you irritable. It will not cause large pimples to populate your face, or make you lose sensitivity in your vulva. Instead, it will improve your overall health and self-esteem.

> "As long as a woman keeps sexually active, it's use it or lose it. Studies have shown that if women have sexual expression either with themselves or with a partner once a week or more, they have twice as much natural estrogen circulating in their body, because you know, you get estrogen from the adrenal glands as well. And also women who maintain sexual activity do not seem to have as much dryness. So there's something that is happening physiologically that needs to be studied because we have not conducted those studies yet."
>
> —Beverly Whipple, The Health Report[7]

Masturbation is a natural painkiller. It can relieve menstrual cramps and migraines (faster than medication), and orgasms may even help prevent endometriosis, a disease of the uterine lining. Jilling off can also make you fall asleep faster, and it can help fire up the immune system to build up resistance to common infections. It can make you happy, reduce stress, and bring self-awareness back to your body and your sexuality. According to a survey of 2,632 women done by sex therapist Carol Rinkleib Ellison, PhD, in which two-thirds of the women had masturbated that month, masturbation was for more than just feel-good fun: 39 percent of the women said it helped them relax, 32 percent said they slept better after masturbating, and 9 percent said masturbation eased their menstrual cramps.[8]

> "When I was around twelve, my mom had a very quick talk with me about how masturbation was okay, and how it was a better choice than having sex with someone else before you were ready. I wasn't brought up to believe that notion of hairy palms and blindness. Those things were like the bogeyman or Satan or something— a made-up scary figure to stop young people from 'unacceptable' behavior."
>
> —Kiley, age twenty-seven

## IT'S OKAY FOR MEN, BUT NOT WOMEN

Our vulvas are not perceived as the veritable pleasure stick his penis is, and therefore we look down at our genitals, literally and figuratively, as if they were second-class citizens to his top dog. Our vulvas don't tell us when they want attention; they don't magically point toward the sky or the ground, or make our pants feel tight all of a sudden. We can't reach out and grab them, and we have to actually figure out what's going on down there by exploring our flaps and folds. We're taught that our vaginas are for making babies and not for sexual pleasure, and nobody teaches us about our clitoris, therefore we believe we're designed to be less sexual than men are. But the truth is, we're not. Sure, we're different than they are—we have monthly cycles and our bodies can more easily align with the moon—but that only goes to prove that our bodies are sacred temples and we need to worship them as such. Some people think that only bad girls masturbate, that nice girls would never do such a thing. But nice girls and bad girls both masturbate, because all women need to revere their bodies, even if we bow down in different ways.

> *"Isn't it interesting that female masturbation was so taboo that the only myths I can think of have to do with men? I feel like men have to masturbate, women don't—that's the difference."*
>
> —Katie, age thirty-two

As we get older, we often become more comfortable in our own skins, more at home in our bodies, more accepting of the sizes and shapes of who we are as women, and more inclined to get to know ourselves better. We discover how we come, and how we don't, and after the first orgasm we want to have more of them. Masturbation allows us the "more" we're looking for without our having to ask anyone else's permission. If he can do it, so can we—and so we should. It doesn't matter if we think of ourselves as bad, good, or somewhere in between. Masturbation doesn't discriminate between boys and girls. No more sexual double standards! No more sluts and studs! Let's get over this hump when it comes to thinking about sex.

## IF YOU DO IT, YOU'RE SELFISH

It's taboo to be selfish. At least, that's how lots of women are co
think. Women are nurturers. We are, or may become, mothers w
of our children, and wives who take care of our partners. And because we're
designated as the homemakers, mothers, and caregivers, our self-love is
often questioned when it should be rewarded, encouraged, and respected.
Traditional values often mean that women are perceived as selfless, as delicate, meek, and loyal. It's hard to feel like the mommy, the caretaker, and
the nurturer and then try to find yourself sexy, independent, and needy. The
combination of the lady and the tramp is difficult for a lot of women to
swallow. But each of us can, and should, be more than one person. We can,
and should, take care of our own needs.

 According to a 2007 Australian study of five hundred women
in their forties, fifties, sixties, and seventies, sexual satisfaction
is strongly associated with good mental health and quality
of life.[9]

If we remain independent, happily unattached, or partnered without marriage or children, we may be thought of as shallow and self-
centered. Community standards tell us that women are supposed to seek
the love of another, and that we aren't complete unless one plus one equals
two. We are supposed to give up our individuality when we enter into a
relationship—as if once we enter the bond of love and/or marriage, we
can't and won't think for ourselves. But as we grow up, we also come to
understand that happiness does not come from somebody else, that we
are responsible for meeting our needs and fulfilling our desires. And more
and more women are throwing out the antiquated ideas associated with
what we should and shouldn't do. We are finding ways to support ourselves financially, emotionally, and sexually. We are searching out orgasms
with and without partners, and we don't expect our partners to teach us

everything we need to know about our sexuality. And this is not selfish. As Betty Dodson once said to me, it's self-full. It is, simply put, sex with oneself. It can improve our relationships, make us better lovers, open us up to new experiences, and allow us to enjoy more of the benefits of partner touch. Masturbation is a teacher, a tool, and a show of appreciation that we do for ourselves. If we don't know how to give love to ourselves, how can we give it to anybody else?

> "I had an abortion when I was seventeen, and that made me feel ashamed and stupid. I blamed myself for everything and was not into sex after that. I became slightly anorexic and very self-conscious around that time, too. But masturbation has helped me overcome my insecurities and my fears, especially from that period. Growing up as a woman affects you in many ways, some you don't even realize, and the pressure is quite brutal from society and family. You need to find your own identity as the woman you will be, and I know that masturbation helped me with that process."
>
> —Salka, age thirty-three

## MASTURBATION IS SECOND-TIER SEX

If we're not the most important people in our lives, then sure, masturbation is not the most important sex we can have. But that's a bah-humbug way to feel about ourselves, don't you agree? So don't think of masturbation like that, either. Masturbation is a great way to address our sexual needs and urges without getting a sexually transmitted infection or having to deal with an unexpected pregnancy. It's pleasure without risk, but that doesn't make it any less satisfactory or any less a sex act than intercourse.

## WHAT IF I BECOME ADDICTED TO MASTURBATION?

If you're like me and go to the gym four or five times a week, you learn to understand the difference between something that makes you feel good and strong and something that makes you feel bad and wrong. An addiction is something you're obsessed with doing, something you can't stop thinking about, to the point where you can't do anything else. If you love masturbating but don't need to do it, if you can go without it for a day, a week, or a month if you must, then you are not addicted. Polishing your pearl is something you can do daily, weekly, or hourly, as long as you still lead a healthy, active life outside of getting off. If you feel yourself thinking up ways to stop functioning in the outside world just so you can touch yourself, then you may have a problem, but before you go cursing the gods, see if you can stop on your own. And once you do, remind yourself that it really isn't a problem at all. As long as it's not affecting your work, your productivity, and your personal life, you'll be A-okay. Here's a personal confession: When I write, I take masturbation breaks. They're sometimes hourly, sometimes daily, and sometimes once every week. The few minutes I allot to masturbation at these times are just what I need to get my endorphins going and bring me back to focusing on my work. I masturbate often, and I feel that there's nothing wrong with masturbation breaks, especially since they help me get back in my game.

> *"If I were a sex educator teaching, I would teach children that masturbation is not wrong. It does not cause you to go blind, does not cause you to go crazy, it does not cause hair to grow on your hands. Our religious leaders have lied about masturbation to our young people for a very long time. Seventy percent of men and women masturbate, and you know, I think it's probably a lot higher than that. The rest lie. So I think we should stop lying to our children."*
>
> —Joycelyn Elders[10]

## MASTURBATION = LOSS OF VIRGINITY

You don't need to save your orgasms until marriage in order to remain a virgin—and besides, what is a virgin, anyway? If you stick a tampon inside of you every twenty-eight days or so, does that make you any less a virgin than if you enjoy rubbing your clit? *Virgin* and *virginity* have come to be relatively subjective terms, but generally a virgin is considered someone who hasn't yet had intercourse with another person. So if this is something you're concerned about, rest assured that masturbating doesn't make you any less a virgin than not doing it. If you've never stuck anything up inside your vagina, and you define virginity as vaginal penetration of any sort, you may want to limit yourself to clitoral stimulation for peace of mind. It's how most women do it anyway, but however you want to do it, you won't deflower yourself if you masturbate.

> *"I wasn't sure for a while if I would ever be able to orgasm with another person, and then later I was unsure that anyone would give me as good an orgasm as I gave myself."*
>
> —Ali, age twenty-four

## EVERYONE WILL KNOW I MASTURBATE

Back when I went to day camp, we used to have this "game" we played where someone would come up behind you and grab at the sides of your body, right above the hips and below the breasts, and pinch your ribs. If you flinched, you weren't a virgin; if you didn't, you were. After flinching the first time, I begged my friends to try again, just to prove to them that the first test was a lie. And even though I knew I was a virgin, there was no way to prove to them, either way, what type of sex I'd had before then. Nobody—no doctor, no teacher, no parent—can tell if you masturbate, or if you've had any other type of sex, unless you go to the doctor with a particular type of sexually transmitted infection or sexually induced inflammation, or if you hang around with evidence, like a vibrator in your pants. There's no test a doctor can administer to tell if you masturbate, and no way for someone to know unless you're caught in the act.

> "My parents didn't talk about masturbation, so it has always been this taboo subject that we weren't supposed to talk about. It's still a taboo subject. I once asked my mom if she could hear anything when I used my vibrators, and she got totally freaked out and couldn't look at me."
>
> —Eleanor, age twenty

And it doesn't matter if your hymen, a layer of mucous membrane surrounding or partially covering the vaginal opening, is or isn't intact. Yeah, lots of girls say when your hymen's broken you're not a virgin anymore, but it's just not true. There are plenty of other easy ways to break your hymen, including using tampons, bicycling, doing gymnastics, and horseback riding. Some women aren't even born with a hymen, and some women have hymens that stretch without tearing. So don't worry if and when you break it; it really has nothing to do with your sexual status. I promise you, your gynecologist will never question the appearance or disappearance of your hymen, and nobody else should, either.

## ONCE YOU'RE IN A RELATIONSHIP, IT'S NOT COOL TO MASTURBATE

Yes, masturbation is solo sex, but that doesn't mean you have to be alone to do it. People without partners do masturbate, but statistics show that women in relationships masturbate more often than their single counterparts, especially women with healthy partnered sex lives. The time you spend alone on yourself is very different from the time you spend focusing on both of you. It's time well spent with yourself, learning things about your own body that your partner may not be able to discover without your help. It's a time when you can focus solely on yourself.

> "Messages of sexuality were very complicated, conflicting, and extremely inappropriate when I was growing up. I was caught masturbating by my stepfather when I was fourteen. As you can imagine, I was absolutely mortified. The incident inspired him to abuse me, and for the next two years I was sexually abused. It's amazing I could ever masturbate again. Therapy was a great help with that. It took me years to regain my sexuality. Thankfully, it is now fully in my possession and I know there's no shame in masturbation or expressing myself sexually."
>
> ——Mischa, age thirty-five

Don't neglect the sensations that occur when you're taking "you" time, and embrace the fact that you can teach your partner a thing or two about your own body. A 2007 study out of Queensland, Australia, showed that 55.2 percent of single women orgasm every single time they masturbate, while only 24.6 percent of women orgasm with a partner.[11] So why deny yourself more orgasms? Besides, women who masturbate are aroused more often than women who don't. Unless you're using masturbation as a crutch and a way to avoid partnersex, it's totally cool to masturbate while you're in a relationship.

## MASTURBATION IS A SIN

In 1975, the Roman Catholic Congregation for the Doctrine of the Faith put out a declaration on sexual ethics that acknowledged that the Catholic Church's stance on masturbation as a mortal sin was often considered antiquated. It went on to acknowledge that psychology and sociology were trying to show that masturbation was a normal part of sexual development—but still, the Vatican's 1976 *Declaration on Certain Questions Concerning Sexual Ethics* continued to look at masturbation as something inherently abhorrent, calling it a "disordered act." The Church reiterated this position in the 1992 *Catechism of the Catholic Church,* but this time the Church agreed to take into account the reasons why people jack or jill off—things like force of habit or mental and social factors—and stated that certain reasons may lessen, or extenuate, a person's guilt from sin.[12]

Lots of Judeo-Christian religious leaders and scholars will tell you that masturbation is not a sin, and most of the more liberal ones, while not actively promoting masturbation, won't spoon-feed you lies about the horrors of doing it. There is nothing in the Bible that specifically says masturbation is a sin. Some sects even promote it as safer sex, and prefer that people choose masturbation over other forms of partnered sex outside of marriage. Touching your own body is your business, and no church, school, or teacher should tell you otherwise.

> *"My parents said practically nothing about masturbation, which I guess is better than saying bad things about it. I went to Catholic school for twelve years but never took the sex part seriously. Most of that time I was an atheist, but every once in a while the idea of an omniscient God peering into my bedroom, watching me masturbate, would creep me out. It added slightly to the hang-up."*
>
> —Mink, age thirty-six

## VULVAS ARE DIRTY

The fact that our genitals aren't external like a penis is means we need to probe around our bodies to figure out how things work. Couple that with the fish jokes, and we learn to think of our vulvas as foul-smelling, dirt-ridden parts of our bodies. We get a lot of negative messages about our genitals from our families and society, including the one where our mothers tell us to make sure we wash "down there," leading us to believe that our natural smell stinks. And then porn shows us that small, tight twats are the perfect pussies, and that if our lips are large and dangly they don't have a chance at the Miss Vulva-verse pageant. The truth is, all vulvas are unique and beautiful. All vulvas are powerhouses of pleasure. The natural pH of your pussy is similar to a glass of red wine's, which means your vulva is slightly acidic, but nothing hard to swallow. You should taste yourself so you know what you taste like, and if you ever think you smell extremely off, odds are, you should check with your doctor. As for how clean our cunts are, the vagina is like one of those self-cleaning ovens: It takes care of itself. You don't need to douche, and you don't need to scrub your vulva with lots of soap. Take care of your body and your body will take care of you.

> *"My older sister told me, 'Hey, if you do this it feels really good.' She didn't show me directly, but she told me if I rubbed myself 'there' really fast, it was really cool. The very first time I came I did it with her in the room (we shared a bedroom). I think she was curious to know if I had the same reaction she did. I don't think I realized it was sexual, per se. We understood it was private, but we didn't understand what an orgasm was. It was just interesting that if you did this, you'd get this really cool feeling. We actually talked about it afterward. There were other times, around that same time in my life, when my girlfriends and I sort of discovered it together, but it was my sister who made me feel like it was normal."*
>
> *—Dusty, age forty-three*

## MY PARENTS SAY IT'S WRONG, OR THEY DON'T SAY ANYTHING AT ALL

Our families, religions, friends, schools, and communities all play a role in how we shape ourselves as individuals. Consciously or subconsciously, what we see, hear, and learn on a daily basis finds a way to sink in under our skin. The thing about older generations is that they were often brought up with a lot less freedom and a lot more fear about all kinds of sexual activity, and many of them therefore don't know how to openly express sexuality to us. This results in a certain way of child rearing that refuses to acknowledge children as sexual beings. We're not taught about sex, gender, or other important parts of how we identify until we've already experienced a lot of anxiety, fear, confusion, and shame over who we are and what we like. What we need to remember is that from infanthood to old age we are all sexual creatures, and we all have the ability to express our sexuality in a number of ways. Masturbation is the easiest way for us to do for ourselves. Our goal may be different when we're young and don't understand orgasm, but it is the one sex act nobody can ever deny us. Odds are, if your parents think it's wrong to masturbate, they have their own issues and discomfort around sex. People spend a lot, or all, of their lives reversing their parents' negative ideas, so instead of letting what your parents think affect your private sex life, let it serve as a reminder to you about how you are different; how you're going to grow up without inhibitions and with loads of orgasms; how you are responsible for your own self; and how you come into this world alone, and you leave alone, and what you do in between is your choice. Maybe when you're comfortable and older, you can talk to your parents about your views, but for now think of yourself, and make sure to show yourself plenty of love.

> *"My parents have wildly different views on sex. My father is a buttoned-down conservative Christian, and thus sex is not a topic we discuss on a regular basis. My mother is a freethinking liberal who is very open about sex. In my later teen years, my mother's attitude helped me deal with my developing sexual desires and changing view of my sexuality."*
>
> —Jay, age twenty

### VIBRATORS DESENSITIZE YOU FOR SEX WITH OTHERS

Vibrators are not a replacement for partners. Instead they are a sexual aid, an enhancement, a way to help you achieve orgasms faster and more often. If you ever feel that a vibrator is coming between you and your partner, talk with him or her about it. If a vibrator helps you achieve orgasm, incorporate the toy into your sex life. If you feel like a vibrator is numbing your clitoris, then stop, relax, and repair. You will not lose sensitivity permanently, if at all, from playing with a buzz on.

> *"I once read that a woman who uses a vibrator will have less enjoyment from sex with a man because she will become too accustomed to the vibrator. Looking back, I wonder if that wasn't written because men were afraid that if women began to enjoy their own orgasms, made for them, by them, men would feel less necessary."*
>
> —Laura, age forty-one

 ## WHEN MASTURBATION ISN'T SO SAFE

There are very few instances when masturbation isn't safe, and most of the "problems" associated with masturbation can be easily remedied by good personal choices and habits. Yes, masturbation is the safest sex you can have, but if you're the kind of woman for whom friction is the name of the game, if you rub too hard you can cause irritation to your clit or the surrounding areas. Intense rubbing for an extended period of time can cause irritation or bleeding, but this discomfort can be altered by changing up your technique or by rubbing more gently. Of course, with excessive rubbing you may need to wait out the chafing, but once you're back to your "regular" self, you'll be just fine to start going at it once again.

Masturbation can also be less safe if you insert dirty things into your vagina. Things like unpeeled bananas or unclean sex toys can lead to other things, like yeast infections and urinary tract infections. To avoid giving yourself an itch, or anything worse for that matter, make sure that all the toys you use are clean, and if you're into fruits, veggies, or other household gadgets, make sure to pop a condom on, or wrap plastic wrap around, the object to keep you safe.

Last, masturbation can be hazardous if it affects your regular productivity or your relationships. If you're finding that you can't carry on with your regular life, if you're forgoing all other types of sex with your partner (that is, if you have a partner), or if you're in a space where you can't think about or do anything outside of masturbating, then you have a problem with the amount of time you devote to masturbation. Still, the risks are few and far between, and odds are, you can find a sacred space in which your self-sexuality can be gratifying, safe, and disease-free.

 ## THINK HAPPY THOUGHTS!

Masturbation is a form of sexual liberation. Women who masturbate have more interest and desire for sex, and when they do have partnered sex, they generally like it more. Women who masturbate have a better self-image and self-awareness and have improved sexual health. When you masturbate you get to control your own desires; you get to drive the car, plan the trip, make the moves. It's all about you.

So how do we move forward toward an enlightened understanding of masturbation without reverting to the negative ideas surrounding self-sexuality? The simple answer is: Permission breeds permission. The more we destigmatize the thought and act of touching our own bodies, the more we give other people permission to do the same. And the more people who get it, who understand that solo sex is not dirty, wrong, or only for losers, the more people will catch on to the fact that it's humanly natural to please ourselves. We have to stop spreading the fear of getting caught and embrace the idea that we want people to know that we tickle our own ivories. So talk to your close friends about doing it, spread the word early on, and make masturbation seem as normal as it is. Know that the reasons people think you shouldn't do it are not valid or truthful, and raise your head high, and place your hand low, and enjoy the freedom to touch your own body.

## DESTIGMATIZING MASTURBATION: ADVICE BY WOMEN, FOR WOMEN

"Do it often—it makes you happy!"
> —*Kryss, age twenty-five*

"Don't worry or be ashamed about where you need to go physically, mentally, or emotionally when it comes to getting off. There's nothing taboo when you're doing it alone and to yourself."
> —*Carrie, age twenty-seven*

"Let your mind run wild."
> —*Tracey, age thirty-four*

"Try doing it while watching an adult movie, or using a toy."
> —*Toni, age thirty-four*

"Experiment! Always experiment!"
> —*Trina, age thirty-six*

"It's all about clit stimulation!"
> —*Eleanor, age twenty*

"Put a small vibrator near the vaginal entrance just when you've brought yourself to orgasm with clitoral stimulation. The feeling of the vibrator there while the muscles contract is amazing."
> —*Jess, age twenty-eight*

"Let yourself laugh or cry afterward. It feels like the ultimate release."
> —*Lauren, age twenty-five*

"Take the time to explore your body."
> —*Suzanne, age twenty-four*

"Think of someone you find attractive, other than the person you're involved with. It turns me on to fantasize without being unfaithful."
> —*Sherry, age thirty-one*

➡

"Remember, no one's watching."
—*Dusty, age forty-three*

"Practice! Practice! Practice! You can't expect to come the first time you masturbate. It takes time to figure out what you like sometimes."
—*Catherine, age twenty*

"Try it with a butt plug. It gives you a much, much more intense orgasm."
—*Natasha, age twenty-three*

"Don't judge! Don't judge yourself, your fantasies, the images that come into your mind as you close your eyes and start touching yourself. And don't judge your partner or his/her fantasies, either. Nothing is dirty or bad or sinful. Whatever brings you joy, pleasure, a great orgasm, as long as it's consensual and no one actually gets hurt, it's all fun and exciting and it's okay!"
—*Candida Royalle, adult film pioneer,*
*Femme Productions*

"Two words: Kegel Exercises. It's all about the Kegel."
—*Jenny, age thirty-six*

"Set your alarm clock for twenty minutes earlier than you normally wake up. When it goes off, pull out your favorite vibe and get off. It's one wake-up call you'll be happy to receive."
—*Caitlin, age twenty-nine*

"As you're about to come, tap on your clit. It brings me to another level."
—*Susan, age twenty-four*

"Do it in the car while your lover is driving. Don't wear panties. Wear a skirt and lift it up and play with your clit while you watch them drive. Tell them their driving turns you on."
—*Tina, age thirty-one*

➡

"Keep an ice cube in your mouth and stick your finger in there so it gets cold. Then place your chilled finger on your clit."
    —*Tania, age thirty-one*

"Do it on the phone. Call your partner and describe, in detail, how you're touching yourself. They'll be over to give you a second orgasm in no time!"
    —*Kal, age twenty-two*

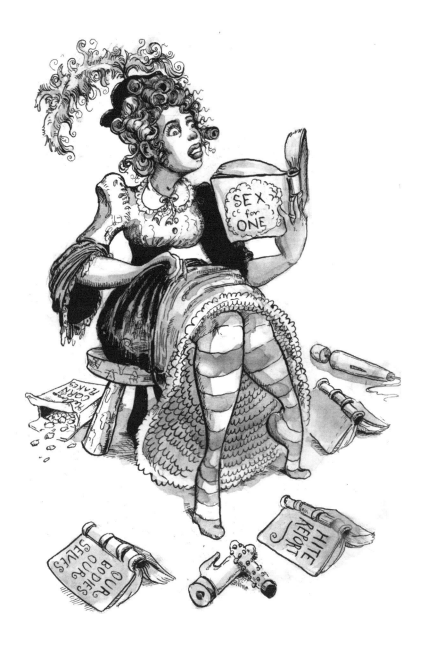

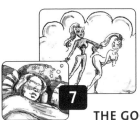

**7**

## THE GOOD, THE BAD, AND THE UGLY:
### *A History of Female Masturbation*

### IN THE BEGINNING

Masturbation wasn't created the way vibrators, butt toys, and porn movies are. It's been around longer than we have, and it will be around long after we're gone. We might not find evolutionary evidence of masturbation in Darwin's teachings, but we can be certain that ever since human beings have had hands, we've found ways to touch and tug, poke and prod, finger and fondle our way through our own intimate folds. Ultrasounds have revealed that masturbation starts in the womb, and in a 1996 letter to the *American Journal of Obstetrics and Gynecology,* several doctors described an ultrasound in which a thirty-two-week-old female fetus used her hand to touch her genitals, focusing mainly on her clitoris. The movements continued on and off for twenty minutes and ended in rapid muscular contractions of her body, followed by relaxation and rest.[1]

Before we know the perceived difference between right and wrong, we just know what feels right. We know how to push our own buttons, the ones that leave us warm and cozy, but that unfortunately, with certain social conditioning, can make us feel wrong and guilty. And we aren't the only animals who do it, either. The bonobo monkeys, among our closest relatives, don't hide their loving feelings when it comes to solo pleasure.[2] Nor does the female porcupine, who will straddle a stick and use it as a sex toy.

Holding on to one end of it with her paws, she'll press the other end against the ground so that it actually vibrates against her genitals.[3]

If we were to travel back in time, to when people lived in tribes—or even caves—to ask our ancestors about masturbation, they'd probably answer us with a simple "Been there, done that." There's proof that over the centuries masturbation has been alternately celebrated, condemned, accepted, and ignored. One of the earliest images of a woman masturbating (a clay figurine) dates back to between 2000 and 4000 BC, and is from the site of an old temple on the island of Malta.[4] And since temples, like our bodies, are places of worship, this is the perfect beginning to the imperfect history of masturbation.

 ## THE GREEKS DID IT WITH DILDOS

The ancient Greeks accepted that sexual pleasure led to sexual health. While one's family and the state were extremely important, the Greeks knew that sometimes you had to take care of yourself. So when it came to female masturbation, the Greeks had the Rolling Stones' "You can't always get what you want, but if you try sometimes, you might find you get what you need" attitude. Dildos, or *olisbos* (taken from the Greek "slip" or "glide"), are talked about as substitutes for sex with their husbands. It was well known that the bustling city of Miletus was home to long and short, wide and narrow, leather and wood, artistic and artificial pricks.

Masturbation wasn't abhorred in Greek culture; it was more or less accepted, especially during war, when men were playing with guns instead of with girls. In Aristophanes' play *Lysistrata*, Lysistrata talks about how sexually frustrated women are during the Peloponnesian war. In another literary fragment by Herodas, two central female characters, Metro and Coritto, discuss their appreciation for both a dildo and its manufacturer. After Coritto receives a bright red dildo from a man named Cerdon, her friend Metro wants to purchase one, too. Comedy ensues as they try to figure out where he lives, and why Coritto didn't buy two dildos instead of one. While this feeds into another of the Greeks' views about oversexed women, it also provides insight into females who are independently sexually fulfilled.[5]

Greek women had the right to be frustrated, both sexually and otherwise. Their husbands weren't always around, and Greek society treated them like second-class citizens whose sole importance was having babies and then taking care of them. In Greek art, women are often seen using instruments of pleasure made out of leather, wood, or ivory to make up for other lost causes.

## MASTURBATION: A SOURCE OF LIFE

Some ancient cultures thought of masturbation as the key to unlocking the flow of energy through the body. They saw masturbation as a way to release the emotions that built up inside our human shells, as well as a way to reconnect with nature. Masturbation was a source of life and a symbol of renewal. The Egyptians wove masturbation into an intricate creation tale. The story goes that their sun god, Atum, literally created the universe through jacking off. Masturbation also bore him children: a son named Shu and a daughter named Tefnut. And how often Atum masturbated determined the tides of the Nile.[6] Unfortunately, while certain civilizations saw masturbation as beneficial to their survival, others did not.

## OH, OH . . . ONAN!

The Bible ignored masturbation, but that didn't stop the story of Onan, in the book of Genesis, from getting appropriated as a cautionary tale against self-love. The story is of a man—actually, he's more of a boy—named Onan who marries his dead brother's wife because his father tells him to. He doesn't necessarily want to marry her, but he has to because it's the law. He knows that when he gets her pregnant, the baby will be considered his dead brother's child. So he decides that he's not going to ejaculate inside her. When he "spills his seed" (really an act of coitus interruptus, rather than an act of masturbation), God kills him.

The irony of this story is that it's used to warn people about the sin of masturbation, but all Onan really did was pull out, and that has nothing to do with masturbation at all. Yet, down the road, onanism and masturbation became somehow related, and they were never completely separated again.[7]

 ## MASTURBATION GONE WILD

The Greek physician Galen believed masturbation was the key to getting rid of excessive bodily fluids and restoring a natural balance to the physical body. He thought women's problems could be resolved if they found a sexual release, and he even encouraged women to masturbate (in limited amounts, because excess was problematic) in order to prevent the so-called "hysterical diseases" brought on by bottled-up sexual tension.[8] His advice remained in use, at times, by doctors treating women with hysteria, but certain physicians, like Nicolas Venette, disagreed with Galen's "buildup and release" technique. Centuries later, in 1696, in his *Tableau de l'Amour Considéré dans l'État du Mariage*, Venette stated that "woman does not have the ability to pollute herself, as does man, or to discharge her superfluous seed. She sometimes retains it lengthily in her testicles or in the horns of her uterus, where it becomes tainted and turns yellow, murky, or foul smelling, instead of white and clear as it was formerly."[9]

## SEPARATION OF CHURCH AND (SOLO) SEX

What makes masturbation so wrong? The truth is, nothing; it's just that masturbation isn't a productive way to procreate, and therefore it in no way benefits the church. Society gives a lot of credence to both sex and religion, so if the two forces stand off against each other, the only way to come out on top is to push every other belief, value, and ideal to the bottom. The beauty of sexuality, though, is that unlike religion it's innate, and nothing we do can stop us from existing as sexual creatures—which is why sex is responsible for many a religious leader's fall from grace. It's something they don't have complete power over. Still, the Church did assert plenty of control, and focused on the guilt and embarrassment of loving thyself; and with that they were successful in making people feel shameful and wrong. And although masturbation has nothing to do with anybody else, and doesn't even involve copulation, it became everybody's business.

Going back to the end of the eleventh century, as part of its reform movement, the Christian Church declared masturbation both vile and evil, and said it was as much a sin against nature as sodomy.[10]

In the thirteenth century, Thomas Aquinas revitalized the sex-negative teachings of Bishop Augustine of Hippo (354–430 CE), who taught that masturbation was one of the most "unnatural sins"—worse than rape, incest, or copulation because it prevented pregnancy from taking place.[11] Later, in the fifteenth century, Jean Gerson, chancellor of the University of Paris and dean of the cathedral school of Notre Dame, spoke out against masturbation. He believed that self-sexuality was the code red of sex because it was both easy to do and easy to keep on doing. Gerson is credited with writing the manuscript "On the Confession of Masturbation," in which he offered priests advice on how to get women and men to confess to what he called "abominable filth" and a "detestable sin."[12]

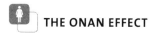

## THE ONAN EFFECT

Somewhere between 1712 and 1716, a long-winded pamphlet called *Onania;* *or, The Heinous Sin of Self Pollution, and All Its Frightful Consequences, in* *Both Sexes Considered, with Spiritual and Physical Advice to Those Who Have* *Already Injured Themselves by This Abominable Practice* was distributed throughout London. The title didn't leave much to the imagination, with the exception of who actually wrote it, and its gospel spread like wildfire. The pamphlet warned masturbators that they would suffer from some serious bouts of horrible illnesses like gonorrhea and epilepsy, and that they would eventually die an early death. It printed what were called "genuine letters" from people who had been inflicted with the sin of masturbation. It told sad stories and provided cures, in the form of a tincture to help strengthen the soul and a powder to help people carry on. In fact, the last part of the book was devoted to these two remedies.[13] It was a brilliant marketing ploy—a way to advertise the aforementioned "medicine," and the perfect scheme for making a menace out of masturbation.

The pamphlet helped feed the minds of people who believed that masturbation was dangerous, and the fear of it was so profitable that doctors and businessmen made sure to jump on the *Onania* bandwagon. This inspired a Swiss doctor by the name of Samuel-Auguste Tissot to publish *L'Onanisme,* a treatise on the disorders produced by masturbation, in the mid-1700s. Tissot believed that most of what *Onania* said was true, and that masturbation was to blame for disease, death, and the bad things that happened to seemingly good people. Aside from the outward symptoms of masturbation—things like loss of memory, loss of strength, sharp pains, pimples, constipation, enlarged clitorises, and hemorrhoids,[14] Tissot also pointed out that female masturbators lacked interest, or were indifferent, when it came to having sex with men.[15] The difference between *L'Onanisme* and *Onania* was that while *Onania* offered a prescription, Tissot discussed the ills of masturbation without marketing any medically available cure. It told readers that masturbation was physically bad for you and should be avoided at all costs, and provided as a cure a healthy diet, pure air, exercise, cold baths, and what Tissot called a "portrait of danger," which brought the masturbator face to face with the terrifying image of their future if they didn't rectify the problem immediately.[16]

Tissot's book became an overnight success. It captured the hearts and minds of all of Europe, and was recognized and referenced by thinkers like Immanuel Kant and Voltaire. Rousseau, too, adored Tissot and felt a kinship with him. Before reading Tissot's work, Rousseau, in his own treatise *Émile*, written to give advice on education, had discussed, in depth, how to discourage young students from masturbating.[17]

In the early 1800s, Goss and Company published the book *Hygeiana*, which stated that girls were as prone as boys, if not more so, to suffering from the dastardly effects of masturbation. The work emphasized the delicacy of women, suggesting that it was this frailty that allowed them to hide their symptoms more easily. Masturbation could lead to "uterine furor," symptoms of which included lackluster lips, a pale complexion, and dulled teeth. Incidentally, these very same symptoms were common in a number of diseases, and therefore it was hard to tell who was touching themselves and who wasn't.[18]

There was good reason to keep masturbation in the realm of the unclean and unsavory. After all, getting people to believe they were wrong if they engaged in it meant money. And the more cures, tinctures, and pills one could pop to prevent visits to "dirty places," the more successes for the doctors promoting these remedies.

Even those for sexual freedom saw masturbation as another beast entirely. One of the best examples of this time is in Richard Carlile's *Every Woman's Book: or, What Is Love?* (1826). While Carlile promoted women's freedom to engage in partnersex, and saw marriage as an undue restraint on sexual passion, he saw masturbation as inherently wrong and dangerous. He placed masturbation along the same lines as pederasty and prostitution, and saw it as the ultimate downfall of the self.[19]

## THE GREAT REPRESSION

During the Victorian era, women were treated as delicate and weak. As a result, general thinking at this time was that frail, vulnerable females would never (gasp!) engage in, or admit to, acts of toxic self-pollution. However, if there was reason to suspect that a woman was endangering her femininity by compromising her position, this situation would be addressed and remedied before she was ruined forever. Thus, the Victorian era, in all its prudish glory, became the era of repression, denial, and sin.

Girls in the Victorian era were restricted from riding horses and bicycles, and later they were forbidden to sew or even to squat down to do laundry, because the feelings associated with these activities could turn a nice girl naughty.

In order to make sure women wouldn't masturbate, the antimasturbation bandwagon continued to churn out speakers and supporters. Dr. Elizabeth Blackwell was one such prominent and outspoken female doctor who espoused the consequences of "bad touch." The first woman MD to graduate from an American medical school, Dr. Blackwell was, needless to say, not a fan of the fingers. In addition to her many accomplishments (including opening the New York Infirmary for Women and Children), she wrote *Counsel to Parents on the Moral Education of Their Children*.[20] In it she discussed controversial topics such as masturbation, which she openly disapproved of, calling it one of the "two vices from which all other forms of unnatural vice springs." She blamed it for domestic violence, and for making both women and men lose their self-control. Still, she was a feminist and a pioneer in her field, and, to her credit, she also claimed that it was wrong to think that women were any less sexual than their male counterparts.[21]

When books, pamphlets, and tinctures didn't stop certain insatiable women, extreme measures could be taken. A well-known London gynecologist/surgeon named Isaac Baker Brown thought that masturbation was the widespread cause of nervous disorders like epilepsy, and further theorized this view in his book *On the Curability of Certain Forms of Insanity, Epilepsy, Catalepsy and Hysteria in Females* (1866). He came up with what he thought was the perfect solution to the imperfection of masturbation. In 1858, he introduced the clitoridectomy, a ferociously cruel way to ensure there were no feel-good effects from touching oneself. It became Baker Brown's signature "quick fix" for the insatiable female, and for years he "successfully" removed the clitoris from an unknown number of women.[22] In 1867, he was banned from the London Obstetrical Society and went insane, and while the clitoridectomy was no longer practiced in Britain, it lived on in the United States well into the twentieth century.[23]

In 1894, Dr. A. J. Block, a physician from New Orleans, shared his disgust over female masturbation in an article entitled "Sexual Perversion in the Female." In it he describes one of his own successes, a case in which a nineteen-year-old girl was cured of a nervous disorder. After Dr. Block manhandled her vagina and labia and found no response, he decided to touch her clitoris. Her body responded with short and rapid breaths, a pale face, and slight moans, and he deduced that the clitoris itself was the cause of her disease and therefore aptly removed it.[24]

In 1868, English psychiatrist Henry Maudsley coined the term *masturbatory insanity* based on the "damage" masturbation caused to the brain.[25] Along those same lines, several gynecologists blamed madness directly on the ovaries. Dr. Robert Battey of Rome, Georgia, was one such example. He operated on women who he felt had no other way out of their miserable existences, and made it his cause célèbre after being deeply affected by the loss of one young female patient whom he thought he could have saved.[26] The operation became known as Battey's Operation, or an ovariotomy, and it involved the removal of both fully functioning, healthy ovaries in order to treat "menstrual madness," nymphomania, and masturbation.[27]

> ## NO MORE CUT CLITS!
>
> It's important to note that while we can scoff at how wrong and absurd mutilation of our genitals sounds, female genital mutilation (FGM), also known as female circumcision and female genital cutting, is still happening in many developing countries around the world. According to the World Health Organization, 80 percent of all FGMs involve removal of the clitoris and the labia minora (inner lips), while 15 percent involve infibulation, which consists of stitching up most of the vagina. FGM is performed for many reasons, including as a social custom, as a way to reduce or eliminate the clitoris in order to reduce sexual desire and enforce virginity, as a cultural identification, for hygienic appeal, and because of myths that enforce the belief that FGMs will enhance fertility and keep children alive longer. It's still practiced in twenty-eight countries in Africa, Asia, and the Middle East. For over 1,400 years, girls and women have been "excised" regularly, and currently the number of women who have undergone FGM is above 140 million. FGM has been acknowledged as a global health problem by the World Health Organization and has been outlawed in the United States only since 1997. While reform is in the works, FGM is still a serious problem in need of attention.[28]

Inhumane practices around masturbation and hysteria continued well into the early 1900s, even as medical opinion and attitudes toward masturbation slowly began to change. In 1936, *Holt's Diseases of Infancy and Childhood* still recommended the cauterization of the clitoris as a way to cure female masturbation.[29]

## CEREAL (ANTI)MASTURBATORS

Two of the most fanatic antimasturbation mavens were men whose lifework continues to impact what we eat for breakfast today. First there was Sylvester Graham (1794–1851), a Presbyterian minister who became well known on the lecture circuit for his "self-pollution" series. Then there was Dr. John Harvey Kellogg (1852–1943), a health nut who received his medical degree from Bellevue Hospital Medical College in New York in 1875. Separately, they worked to change the nation's diet and sexual appetite.

Sylvester Graham preached about the simplicity with which one could spot a victim of self-abuse. Describing a masturbator in detail, he explained how they were introverted, unclean, and tired, and had lots of acne or other skin problems. They would grow up with cancerous lesions, and die a slow and painful death. While Graham eventually moved away from his masturbation rhetoric and began focusing more of his attention and affection on his nutritional plan for a healthy, happy life, he never lost interest in condemning the abominable sin. His focus on healthful eating led him to theorize that the world would be a much-improved place if everybody understood the negative effects of eating (and beating) their meat. His theory said that meat eaters lusted after more in life, desired further vices, and therefore were more prone to abusing their bodies. To further exemplify his teachings, he preached that married couples should practice excessive sexual moderation, meaning sex no more than once a month.

Dr. John Harvey Kellogg admired Graham, and when he had his chance, as the staff physician at the health reform institute known as Battle Creek Sanitarium (or "the San"), he also promoted a strict regime of bland foods and daily exercise. Kellogg, too, believed that the key to being fit entailed sexual starvation. He thought masturbation was the most dangerous of the sexual behaviors, and in his *Treatment for Self-Abuse and Its Effects* he described numerous ways to stop children from getting off. His treatments included tying a masturbator's hands together and circumcising a male without anesthesia (so that he remembered the pain). For women, Kellogg had another suggestion: to pour a bit of pure carbolic acid, a toxic liquid and disinfectant also known as phenol, directly on the clitoris, burning it so badly that no woman would ever want to touch there again. Kellogg performed at least one clitoridectomy, on a ten-year-old girl whose father was certain that she would be damned if drastic measures were not taken.[30]

This was a man who spent the first night of his honeymoon writing his *Plain Facts for Old and Young*, a 644-page treatise with a 97-page focus on masturbation. He claimed that a masturbating woman was likely to suffer from nervous exhaustion and emaciation, as well as flat-chestedness, memory loss, fickleness, and an irritable disposition. And these were only a few of the thirty-nine symptoms and effects masturbation might impart.[31]

Kellogg also believed that a child should be served cold, instead of hot, cereals at breakfast, in order to quell the child's masturbatory urges. And eventually, like Graham, he created his own signature food designed to curb masturbation and sexual desires. That's how graham crackers, and later cornflakes, came to be—though that's not why people eat them today, since Graham and Kellogg would never have approved of certain ingredients, like refined flour and sugar, used in their modern-day products.[32]

 Between 1856 and 1932, the U.S. Patent Office handed out thirty-three patents to the inventors of antimasturbatory devices.[33]

 ## SELF-LOVE AND LOATHING: STRAIGHT FROM THE PSYCHE

At the end of the nineteenth century, the British sexologist Havelock Ellis released his *Studies in the Psychology of Sex: The Evolution of Modesty; the Phenomena of Sexual Periodicity; Auto-Erotism*. In the first volume of his seven-volume *Studies*, Ellis publicly laid into Tissot and his congregation of loyal disciples. Ellis suggested that moderate masturbation was a healthy way to relieve stress and calm the nerves, though he also warned that too much masturbation could lead to slight, yet harmful, problems associated with the skin, digestion, and circulation.[34] Ellis was the man who coined the word *autoeroticism,* and, although he didn't believe that masturbation would harm children, he thought that young adults who masturbated became horribly self-conscious and insecure because they lacked the physical affection and attention that came from being with another human being. He also believed that excessive masturbation was the main cause of divorce for intelligent women, since it gave them an aversion to "normal" coitus.[35]

Other doctors, like Dr. John Meagher, saw masturbation as far worse for women than for men, and called it socially unacceptable for a married woman to masturbate. Meagher thought women might be using it as a form of birth control, and that this would indeed lead to disorders of the nervous system. He saw it as a rejection of other forms of coitus,[36] as did the conservative critic Walter Gallichan. Saying that women often preferred masturbation to sex, Gallichan described the act as "blunting the finer sensibilities" when it came to sex in marriage.[37] But other sexologists, like Magnus Hirschfeld, Wilhelm Stekel, and Alfred Kinsey, were starting to change how people thought about masturbation. And in 1950, thirty years after it was first published in German, Wilhelm Stekel's book *Auto-Eroticism* was translated into English. In it, Stekel examines masturbation as universal and natural, and says the problems around masturbation arise when other people start meddling with the affairs of one's hand.[38]

There were also women like Stella Browne, a socialist and sexual radical, who thought masturbation was the fine line between promiscuity and celibacy, and advocated for the use of hands in order to maintain a wellbalanced society.[39] And slowly but surely, masturbation became seen as an act of independence and an ideal way for women to take sexual matters into their own hands.

**FREUD AND THE FEMALE**

Austrian neurologist Sigmund Freud, like Ellis, thought masturbation was a narcissistic act. He believed masturbation created a fantasy life that was an ill substitute for reality, and that could bring on antisocial behavior and psychic problems. He viewed masturbation as the transitional stage between childhood and adulthood, and saw it as a way for the body to train for its more important, and more mature, journey toward heterosexuality.

Freud wasn't gung ho about going downtown by oneself, but he didn't necessarily think of masturbation as a disease of the body; he saw it more as a disease of the mind. He believed that jilling off should be done sparingly, to ensure that neurotic, overly sensitive females didn't lose their minds. He felt masturbation was more unnatural in women than in men, and even referred to it as a masculine activity. On top of all this, he emphasized the importance of vaginal orgasms over clitoral ones, calling vaginal orgasms the more mature orgasms. Freud believed that women needed to outgrow masturbation in order to fully appreciate and enjoy penetrative sex. The end of masturbation (clitoral stimulation) signified the beginning of the mature sexual development that made a girl a woman. Freud did acknowledge that masturbation had its benefits as a major stress reliever, and as a way to avoid sexually transmitted infections, but he also warned of its negative psychological effects and believed that it could reduce sexual potency.[40]

While it's been years since Freud's "findings" have affected our teachings on masturbation, his work was such a critical component of our understanding of modern psychology that it took years for women (and doctors) to understand that the clitoral orgasm was not the immature predecessor of the vaginal orgasm. We now know that lots of women need some form of clitoral stimulation to get off, even with vaginal penetration.

Masturbation as a "functional and nervous disorder" was finally removed from *Holt's Diseases of Infancy and Childhood*, a well-known pediatric textbook, in 1940. *Holt's also* no longer recommended restraints, reprimands, or surgery as means of curbing masturbation. Instead, the authors wrote that masturbation didn't actually cause physical harm, even though it could cause emotional embarrassment and guilt.[41]

 ## THE KINSEY EXPERIMENT

In 1947, in middle America, Alfred Kinsey became the pioneering force behind a new sexual movement. A biologist, professor of both zoology and entomology, and founder of the (Kinsey) Institute for Research in Sex, Gender, and Reproduction at Indiana University, Kinsey was an openly bisexual man whose mission was to change people's perceptions of sex. He first reported on men's sexual behavior in his 1948 *Sexual Behavior in the Human Male*, a work that was widely acknowledged and accepted. However, in 1953, when he published arguably the most comprehensive (and important) study on female sexuality, the general public was less forgiving. Across America, church leaders and other educators labeled his findings amoral and against family values.[42] Senator Joseph McCarthy even went so far as to call it communism.[43] Though Kinsey lost the support of the Rockefeller Foundation because of the controversy, his work was still groundbreaking. In his *Sexual Behavior in the Human Female* survey, women not only walked the walk, they talked the talk—about sex and masturbation.

So what did he reveal about masturbation? Kinsey described masturbation as an essential outlet for the pre–*Sex and the City* girl, but topped it off by mentioning that it was also extremely valuable for married women. Of the 5,940 women interviewed for his survey, 62 percent actually masturbated, with 58 percent reaching orgasm—a much higher percentage than had ever admitted to doing so before. The average time to orgasm during self-love was less than three minutes. And masturbation, Kinsey noted, provided 7 to 10 percent of all orgasms in women ages sixteen to forty.[44]

As is the case with any research, some of Kinsey's findings were biased. For starters, his study sample was made up almost entirely of middle-class, college-educated, under-thirty-five white adults, who represented a small sampling of the population. Some of his methods for interviewing have also been questioned. And since Kinsey was so out about his own alternative lifestyle, his work might not reflect the sentiments of a larger, more conservative population. His research continues today through the Kinsey Institute in Indiana, and through the work of sex therapists, educators, and researchers around the world.

##  DR. MASTERS AND MS. JOHNSON

Dr. William H. Masters was a physician with a piqued interest in the experience of sex, and in 1957 he hired a research assistant by the name of Virginia Johnson, whom he later married (and, even later, divorced), to help him forge ahead in exploring the topic. Masters and Johnson actually observed people having sex, both solo and partnered, and were responsible for turning sex therapy into a legitimate, commercial, and profitable occupation. In their 1982 book *Human Sexuality* (cowritten with Dr. Robert Kolodny), they devote a chapter to solitary sexual behavior, and call masturbation "the ultimate source of our sexual self-awareness." They endorse masturbation as a way to alleviate problems like anorgasmia (the inability to reach orgasm), stress, and insatiable sex drives.[45]

Despite all this proactive thinking about masturbation, certain religious institutions still clung to their outdated beliefs that masturbation was an "intrinsically and seriously disordered act."[46] Not to be deterred, Masters and Johnson continued, along with Kinsey, to be driving forces in sex research worldwide.

In 1972, the American Medical Association concluded that masturbation was a normal sexual activity.[47]

## REACHING NEW HITES

When Shere Hite published her groundbreaking 1976 study on female sexuality, she gave women their "sex voice," allowing them to speak openly about their own sexual experiences and desires. Instead of actually observing how they did it, like Masters and Johnson did in their study, Hite asked women to describe their experiences. Three thousand women responded to *The Hite Report,* answering questions on everything from masturbation to sexual slavery to partnersex and the sexual revolution. When it came to solo sexploration, Hite's research revealed that 82 percent of women had tried masturbation.[48]

Her work was essential because it was the first comprehensive study on female sexuality published by a woman for other women. It allowed women to speak in their own words about who they were sexually. Hoping to redefine female sexuality by giving the general public a new perspective, Hite also provided insight into the more complex thoughts of women.

## A ONE-WOMAN MASTURBATION MACHINE

Myriad women love masturbation, thanks to Betty Dodson and her one-woman campaign to take back the female hand job. *Liberating Masturbation: A Meditation on Selflove* (it later became *Sex for One* when she sold it to Crown Publishing in 1986) was Dodson's first book on the subject. Published in 1974, it provided women with the details, freedom, and fuel they needed to feel good about taking back their sex lives. Its success was stupendous. Dodson sold 150,000 copies without a distributor, and since its 1986 publication, *Sex for One* has sold over one million copies worldwide.

Dodson, a talented and classically trained fine artist, grew up in the Bible Belt of Kansas and made her way east at the young age of twenty. In New York, she developed a slide show called *Creating an Aesthetic for the Female Genitals,* which showcased the beautiful world of the female organ. Loaded with a bag of sex toys and one hundred color slides of female genitalia, Dodson first introduced her show at the 1973 NOW sexuality conference in New York City. Over one thousand women showed up to watch slide after slide of various vulvas.

Dodson began masturbating at an early age, and took her first peek between her thighs at the age of ten. What she saw shocked her. Her inner lips weren't perfect, and her labia, as she described them, "were the same funny-looking things that dangled from a chicken's neck."[49] Blaming their appearance on masturbation, she thought she had ruined her genitals and subsequently swore off solo sex. The ban didn't last long (a few days), and through her fine art and her perseverance, Dodson has been teaching women how to love their bodies ever since.

## THE RISE OF THE FEMINIST SEX SHOPS

In 1974 Dell Williams, a former actress and advertising account executive, began selling sex toys to women through her mail-order business, Eve's Garden, in New York. She set up a boutique in a small showroom on the fourteenth floor of a Manhattan office building, empowered by the belief that orgasmic women could create global change.

Out West, Joani Blank was starting her own sexual revolution. A sex educator and author, she was looking for a place to distribute her work when she founded the sex-toy shop Good Vibrations in 1977. Good Vibrations was not only the first female-owned and operated sex-positive sex store on the West Coast, but it was also a haven for feminist activity and information. Blank knew that sex wasn't just about fun, and that it had political value as well. So, while she was all about promoting healthy sexuality, especially masturbation, she also felt the need to create a "clean, well-lit sex store" as a sanctuary for women (and men who weren't into the typical "adult" store experience). With a predominantly female workforce trained to educate customers, and stores that were comfortable for people of all sexual orientations and lifestyles, Good Vibrations set the bar high for other types of sex-positive shopping experiences. Now there are over a dozen similar sex stores across North America, and even in Europe. They often allow you to handle (as in touch, not use) sex toys before you make a purchase.

 ## MASTURBATION IN THE '90S

In 1993, Samuel and Cynthia Janus, who together compiled their research and published *The Janus Report on Sexual Behavior,* noted that 38 percent of women masturbated on a regular basis, compared with 55 percent of men. Eleven percent of women said they never masturbated.[50] The following year, additional studies were done uncovering more of the sexual climate in America. The first was a survey of 647 never-married female undergraduate students from a residential Midwestern university. Of the 647 women, only 16.3 percent admitted to masturbating.[51]

A larger, more comprehensive study from 1994 was *Sex in America.* Drawing on a random sampling of 3,432 respondents, the study's four researchers explored several assumptions about masturbation. Forty percent of the females in the study had masturbated at least once that year, and the majority of those women were in their thirties. The study concluded that 45 percent of women who masturbated were white, college-educated, sexually experimental women who lived with a partner. The research also indicated that "the practice (of masturbation) is so strongly influenced by social attitudes that it becomes more of a reflection of a person's religion and social class than a hidden outlet for sexual tensions."[52]

## TO INFINITY AND BEYOND

In the past few years, the popularity of pleasure parties has grown tenfold. Women now meet to share drinks, conversation, and sex toy advice in living rooms around the country. They talk about how to use sex gadgets, both alone and with a partner. And because they purchase their products in the security of someone's home, they feel less shameful about doing it. In a way, they are bringing back the *Sex and the City* mentality of girl talk. And talking leads to knowledge, which leads to better sex.

It could be a sign of the times, or maybe it's just about time, but masturbation has become a part of a woman's complete sexual experience. Masturbation has come to signify sexual liberation, independence, and the acceptance of the free-to-be-you-and-me mind-set. Sex toy companies, adult videos, artists, and feminists have all found ways to showcase masturbation as a positive outlet for both body and mind.

Masturbation, while still something to do in private, has finally gained a public forum. Some women and young girls now get their masturbation tips and techniques from girlie magazines that rely on either reader surveys or hired writers to dish masturbatory dirt. Others get their information online, in chatrooms or from websites. But, even though it feels like female orgasms are on the rise, masturbation remains on the down-low.

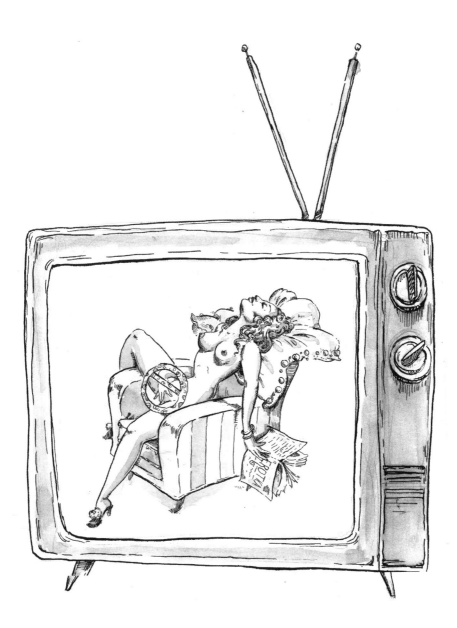

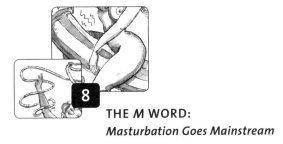

## 8

## THE *M* WORD:
### *Masturbation Goes Mainstream*

> *"People, and most magazines and books giving sexual advice, do not talk about masturbation in the same way they talk about orgasms or oral sex. Masturbation remains in the shadows, a practice that few discuss."*

—*Sex in America: A Definitive Survey*[1]

WHERE DO WE GET THE LOWDOWN on going down on ourselves? Who teaches us about solo sex, and how do we spread the gospel of self-love? Where are our images about masturbation coming from? What are magazines and television saying to us about self-pleasure? When it comes to guys wanking off, you'll find mentions of it on late-night TV, on comedy channels, and in repeat episodes of the new *Battlestar Galactica,* but you'd be hard pressed to find the same types of mentions when it comes to women loving themselves.

The last great sex survey, *Sex in America,* was done in 1994, a time when 40 percent of all the eighteen- to fifty-nine-year-old women questioned admitted to having masturbated at least once in that very same year. Of the 40 percent of wankettes, only one in ten admitted to petting the kitty weekly. Another 50 percent of women said that they never masturbated, ever.[2] Now, if we were to jump back eighteen years, to 1976, we would find that, according to *The Hite Report*, a whopping 82 percent of women masturbated. So what's going on here? Are fewer of us doing it, or are fewer of us talking about what we're doing? Is masturbation going the way of the dinosaur, or is it secretly soaring behind closed doors?

> *"While it is rather common for men to talk and joke about masturbation, it is another thing for women to do so. For some reason women do not admit as freely to masturbation as men. I followed a recent chat board discussion among teenaged girls at a website where I volunteer and they all agreed that expressing their sexual confidence was something they found challenging. They could talk about sex in general or about partnered sexual activities, but talking about solo sex was almost taboo. So there still remains some shame about sex with the younger generation. We have come a long way when it comes to talking candidly about sex but there are still some boundaries we have not overcome."*
>
> —*Seska Lee, Seskuality.com*[3]

Here's the first problem: Unless you interview every woman in the United States, which is impossible, you do not know how many women actually masturbate and how many women don't. Even then, you can't guarantee that people won't lie when it comes to questions about such a personal topic. And no matter who's doing the research, all surveys are essentially flawed because they're being answered by only a small percentage of any given population. Both *The Hite Report* and *Sex in America* surveyed upwards of three thousand people and based the results of their surveys on this population. Now, granted, when it comes to how to masturbate, there is, for most of us, a more limited means to an end, at least in terms of technique; but when it comes to who does and doesn't masturbate, that's a very individual thing. Just because one mother in Iowa says she would never masturbate doesn't mean another mother in Iowa feels the same way. People who answer most surveys may also be self-selecting, and I wouldn't be surprised if the women who responded to these sex surveys were women with strong convictions about sex, especially female sexuality.

So why is it that in 2007 masturbation, while practiced by many, is talked about by few? Not all women proudly admit that they stroke one out. Some women would rather talk about getting fucked by their boy-friends or fingered by their girlfriends than about masturbation, even if self-love gives them the best orgasms of their lives. We lose some of our dependence on relationships if we admit that we know our bodies best, and so we often choose to hand that ownership over to some other indi-vidual just so we can show that we play well with others. If we double-click our mice better than our partners do, we may feel guilt and sadness about not being able to translate that into our "other" sex life. Some people don't even consider masturbation sex, or they call it lesser sex. But masturba-tion is sex, and it's some of the best sex out there. It's sex without trying to procreate; it's self-full sex; and it's definitely the safest sex you can have (assuming that you are not going to get crazy and stick an unpeeled fruit up your vagina or use a sharp object on your clit). Getting off alone is about achieving orgasm, or at least a state of ecstatic being, without anybody else's love, help, or presence (though with mutual masturbation, somebody else is physically present, of course). Because of its truly solitary nature, not enough women want to admit that they could be so selfish as to choose to love themselves. The time to stop caring about what other people think is now. Start spreading the *M* word, loud and proud.

> *"I hang out with a bunch of really politicized women who identify as feminist and who write and publish sex-positive work and talk a big masturbation-is-healthy-and-good talk in the sense of reporting on other people's art about it, publicizing research that shows the benefits, et cetera. Yet I've never had a really good, long, detailed, personal conversation with one of them about it. It still feels like there's some shame or silence about it. I do think there's been some progress, but I also think we've mistaken a highly normative, commoditized sex culture for a diverse, queer, liberated sexual agency. Especially for women, I think we're far from living in a culture that views and supports our sexuality in a healthy, complex, non-normative way."*
>
> —Kovner, age twenty-eight

##  BOYS VS. GIRLS

A boy has a penis that dangles on the outside of his body from the day he's born. It's something he can grab, pull, tug, and touch without anybody having to explain anything to him. Women don't have that luxury. It's just not the same if we grab, pull, or tug at our vulvas. For most of us, the process of figuring out what feels good, including finding our clit in the first place, takes a lot of work and effort. This means that not only do boys have it easier, but it's also more acceptable and understandable that they masturbate. They don't have to dig inside to find what they're looking for; it's been laid out in a nice package and presented to them at birth. Girls have to find and then unwrap their surprise.

So when it comes to explaining masturbation, it's so much easier for a guy to express himself. Growing up, we all quickly learn what it means to see a boy moving his open fist up and down in front of his body. When we "get with the program," we know he's gesturing a universal symbol for male masturbation. Guys can jack off, whack one out, choke the chicken, or pull their chain. Women don't have that same vocabulary to express their sexuality. In fact, most of the female terms for masturbation may be funny, but a lot of them are also insulting. Which proves the point that—as a society—we're not all that comfortable with women masturbating.

> "I learned to be curious about masturbation from two of my closest friends. They asked me if I did it, told me how they did, and encouraged me to try. One of them even bought me my very first vibrator. So is that a product of me just growing up, or is it indicative of some bigger paradigmatic shift?"
>
> —Melissa, age twenty-six

## JILLING OFF and OTHER TERMS for FEEL-GOOD FUN[4]

- A night in with the girls
- Auditioning the finger puppets
- Banging the box
- Beating around the bush
- Buttering the muffin
- Checking the oil
- Cleaning between the camel's toes
- Cleaning your fur coat
- Coaxing the turtle out of her shell
- Cunt-cuddling
- Digging in
- Diving for pearls
- Doodling the noodle
- Double-clicking the mouse
- Driving Ms. Daisy
- Dunking your doughnut
- Entering the forest

➡

- Exploring the bush
- Fanning the fur
- Finding yourself
- Finger-banging
- Finger painting
- Flicking the switch
- Fucking without complications
- Genital manipulation
- Getting a lube job
- Getting in touch with the man in the boat
- Getting to know yourself
- Going solo
- Having sex with someone you love
- Hitchhiking south
- Jilling off
- Joycelyn Eldering
- Letting your fingers do the walking
- Ménage à moi
- Mistressbating
- Pearl-diving
- Petting the kitty
- Playing the slots
- Polishing your pearl
- Practicing safe sex
- Putting the dot in (dot)org
- Ringing the bell
- Rocking the boat
- Rubbin' Hood
- Shebopping
- Spanking the spot
- Surfing the channel
- Taking a dip
- Taking advantage of yourself
- Tending to your garden
- Tickling your fancy
- Tiptoeing through the two-lips
- Touching your tigress
- Twinkling your little star
- Walking downtown
- Whipping your cream

## CELEBRITIES WHO "LOVE" THEMSELVES

Pop icons like Madonna and Britney Spears really know how to piss people off, and one way they've done it is by mentioning masturbation. In 1990, the Pope asked his followers to boycott Madonna's *Blonde Ambition* tour because, among other things, she simulated masturbation onstage. Yep, that's right—during her rendition of "Like a Virgin," Madonna pretended to masturbate. The police in Toronto threatened to arrest her and charge her with indecency if she didn't change her performance. Madonna didn't change a thing, though, and the show went on as planned (you can see the occurrence in her 1991 documentary, *Truth or Dare*). In 1993, Madonna did it again on the big screen in the movie *Body of Evidence*. In the movie, her character was overtly sexual, which served as some sort of justification for her character's explicit masturbation, which again supports the perceptions of the type of woman who masturbates.

Britney Spears had the ovaries to discuss masturbation in a 2003 interview with *People*. Spears is quoted as saying, "I think if you say you don't do [masturbation], you're lying. It's a positive thing to indulge in. I don't do it all the time. It's life. Guys can talk about it. Why can't girls? I think it's positive for girls not to depend on guys."[5] The once-virginal Spears (virgins can and should masturbate, by the way) encouraged girls to masturbate and to spread the gospel of self-love. Spears's declaration of self-love made international headlines, more likely for its supposed "shock value" than for its positive message.

And whether Madonna and Brit spoke up out of courage or just to provoke, no one bats an eye when it comes to men jacking off. (Though admitting one does it and getting caught are entirely different things.) When famous masturbator Paul Reubens, a.k.a. Pee-wee Herman, a children's TV host and comedian, was arrested for masturbating in an X-rated movie theater, the public perception of masturbation sank to an all-time dirty low. But still, it was more that he did it in public than that he did it at all. When

Prince simulated masturbation on his guitar at the halftime show for the 2007 Super Bowl, reactions ranged from surprise to amusement to total complacency. Still, there were few complaints, and it was barely an item in the papers the next day.[6] Janet Jackson, however, did not fare so well. When her breast was outed after an unfortunate "wardrobe malfunction" a few years prior, it was not as easy to dismiss and move on.

Men are considered wankers by birth, while women are considered wanking material by birth, but we're not necessarily seen as wankers in our own right. The truth is, we are strokettes and we will continue to grope ourselves when we're alone. And we'll gossip about getting off in small, safe groups, even if we sometimes look to props to make us more comfortable talking about it in public. In fact, lots of female celebrities have commented on their love of sex toys, more than have commented on their love of manual stimulation. Madonna used sex toys in her book *Sex*. Roseanne Barr told the MTV Video Music Awards that Hitachi made such good vibrators, she was going to buy herself one of their TVs. Actress Anne Heche happily promotes her love for vibrators: "Vibrators are great—they save people from having stupid sex. I'd pitch them to anybody." Hip-hop artist Missy Elliott sang the praises of her favorite kind of vibe in her hit song "Toyz." After her divorce, Halle Berry was spotted at a West Hollywood sex shop, the Pleasure Chest. She later told Handbag.com, "You can't forget your sexuality. You can still embrace your body by going to the gym or going to [a sex shop]."[7] In December 2004, *Desperate Housewives* star Eva Longoria told *Rolling Stone* about the best sex she'd had all year. It was "probably with my vibrator. I own two. I have the rabbit one, and I give that as a gift all the time. To other girls. For a birthday or the like. It's the best gift to give: an orgasm. And if I can't do it for ya, I'll give you the tools to succeed! I have one rabbit and a Pocket Rocket."[8] Longoria's costar Teri Hatcher told *Harper's Bazaar* that she had a lot of sex with her vibrator, and that it kept her happy in her single life.

## CAUGHT on CAMERA: FEMALE MASTURBATION on the BIG SCREEN

LOOKING FOR INSPIRATION? CHECK OUT THIS SELECT GROUP OF SOLO-SEX SCENES:

*BODY DOUBLE* (1982) Melanie Griffith plays a porn star famous for her masturbation scenes.

*LIKE WATER FOR CHOCOLATE* (1992) Gertrude (Claudette Maillé), the main character's sister, has to find a way to release herself after a particularly arousing meal.

*SINGLE WHITE FEMALE* (1992) Jennifer Jason Leigh plays a psychopath who makes love to her mattress in this suspense-filled thriller.

*THE SLUMS OF BEVERLY HILLS* (1998) Natasha Lyonne takes her cousin's vibrator for a test-drive in a hot and funny solo-sex scene.

*MULHOLLAND DRIVE* (2001) Before Naomi Watts did *King Kong*, she masturbated in this creepy David Lynch film.

*SECRETARY* (2002) This flick is hot, and heavy on the kink, and Maggie Gyllenhaal gives a standout solo performance.

*SLACKERS* (2002) Laura Prepon (Donna from *That '70s Show*) is interrupted while masturbating with a huge dildo. Even though another character forgets to knock, Prepon carries on, asking him to leave so she can finish what she started.

*THE OH IN OHIO* (2006) Parker Posey plays a woman on a mission. Trying to achieve her first orgasm, she goes at it in a variety of ways in this lighthearted, comedic attempt at reaching one's peak.

*RABBIT FEVER* (2006) This British mockumentary is all about the Rabbit vibrator and the effects of its popularity on regular society. The humorous focus is on Rabbit addicts who are trying to kick their addiction.

Of course, vibrators also keep married women satisfied. There's the story of soccer star David Beckham buying his wife, Posh Spice, a $1.8 million diamond-encrusted vibrator.[9] Jenny McCarthy, former *Playboy* bunny and actress, told talk-radio host Howard Stern that her favorite vibe was the Pocket Rocket, and that she used it more than once a week. Incidentally, I bought my first vibe in 1996 after listening to Howard Stern talk about his ex-wife Alison's love of the Pocket Rocket. I thought, *If Howard's wife can use a vibrator, then so can I.* Howard Stern's discussion of his now-ex-wife's Pocket Rocket is a perfect example of the power of celebrity. I don't know if I would have bought a vibrator that day, or even that year, if I hadn't heard Stern say it was okay. No one had ever told me it was okay, or fun, to use a sex toy before. In fact, as soon as I came, I called my girlfriends and told them they all had to try it, too. The point is, the more celebrities positively promote self-sexuality, the more likely the word, and the deed, are to spread.

## LITERARY SMUT

D. H. Lawrence, the twentieth-century writer, may have been the first person to give a description of female masturbation in his book *The Rainbow*. Though Lawrence merely alludes to the character Anna's moments of self-pleasure, calling them a "dance" that she does in secret, it was quite radical at the time of its publication. Lawrence was criticized many times over the course of his life for being lewd, obscene, and sex-crazed. When *The Rainbow* came out in 1915, it was deemed obscene and all copies of it were seized and destroyed in Britain.

Decades later, Erica Jong's 1973 novel *Fear of Flying* also caused quite a stir. Called the female version of *Portnoy's Complaint* (Philip Roth's 1969 novel about the character Alexander Portnoy's guilt, shame, and high sex drive), it's where the term *zipless fuck* (a sexual encounter without commitment or emotional involvement) comes from, and, although it was a novel, it was also a book that encouraged women to masturbate. Jong told the

United Kingdom's *Guardian*, "I know that psychiatrists were recommending the book to female patients. There were so many women then who couldn't fantasize or masturbate because they were so uptight, and here was a book that said, go ahead."[10] Jong's main character, Isadora, masturbates, and her self-love activity is written with descriptive language that includes a mention of her clitoris. Critics were both amazed and appalled at Jong for being so honest about female sexuality[11]—for depicting a woman not only having sex, but liking it, and admitting to masturbation. Thirty-some years later, the book has sold over twelve million copies worldwide.

---

### SONGS FOR STROKING

All of these songs have two things in common. First, they're all performed by women. Second, they intentionally, if not overtly, discuss masturbation.

"Cumming into My Own," by the Lunachicks
"Fingers," by Pink
"First Orgasm," by the Dresden Dolls
"Forgiven," by Alanis Morissette
"Handyman," by Joan Jett and the Blackhearts
"Icicle," by Tori Amos
"I Don't Need a Man," by the Pussycat Dolls
"I Touch Myself," by the Divinyls
"Right in Time," by Lucinda Williams
"Sat in Your Lap," by Kate Bush
"She Bop," by Cyndi Lauper
"Sleep Forever," by Bree Sharp
"Take Care," by Janet Jackson
"Too Much of You," by Kelly Osbourne
"Touch Myself," by T-Boz
"Touch of My Hand," by Britney Spears
"Toyz," by Missy Elliott
"Vibe On," by Dannii Minogue
"Wiggley Fingers," by Patty Griffin
"You're Makin' Me High," by Toni Braxton

This was not how it played out for author Judy Blume. She first wrote about masturbation in her young adult book *Deenie* (1973), the story of a teenage girl with scoliosis. Because of what Blume wrote, *Deenie* has been banned more than any other Blume books. The line that most frequently gets *Deenie* in trouble is: "[That week] I touched my special place practically every night. It was the only way I could fall asleep and besides, it felt good."[12] Blume wrote the scenes based on her own experiences, and has been quoted as saying, "Masturbation is such a frightening idea to some adults, they would rather ban a book than talk to their children about it. Sad for their kids."[13]

> *"I remember when the song 'I Touch Myself' came out and not being really sure what she meant, but knowing it was intriguing. I never had 'the talk.' I don't even know how I learned about sex."*
>
> —Katie, age thirty-two

 ## TUNING THE KNOB: MASTURBATION ON TV

In 1992, a radical breakthrough was made on prime-time television when masturbation became the focal point for a whole episode of "must-see TV." When the popular television show *Seinfeld* debuted its episode "The Contest," masturbation became a sport, a sort of acknowledged national pastime. The specific episode pitted the four main characters against each other in a competition to see who could go the longest without self-pleasure. In stereotypical fashion, the men all agreed that masturbation was more critical to the male lifestyle than to the female one, and allowed Elaine to participate only if she placed a higher wager on the (lack of) action. Elaine was, ironically, the second to fold, driving home the point that women masturbate too. Interestingly, the NBC censors would not allow the word *masturbation* to be used in the episode, so the term *master of your domain* became its replacement. Since then, it's become common social slang for the deed.[14]

There have been other references to masturbation in *The Family Guy, The Simpsons, Futurama, That '70s Show, Roseanne*, and *Saturday Night Live.* With the exception of *SNL*'s, all these references regard male masturbation. The most significant and powerful representation of female sexuality to ever air on national television happened on cable. That's where four women met weekly to talk about shoes, secrets, and the search for love. The show was called *Sex and the City*, and it progressively changed people's perceptions of women's wants and needs. Premiering on June 6, 1998, *Sex and the City* tackled feminist issues and other social, cultural, and sexual problems through the eyes of four women in their thirties and forties. As the title suggests, the episodes were dedicated to all things sex, with masturbation appearing more than once over the show's six-year life span. From discussions of masturbation fantasies to the famous episodes of vibrational exploits with the Rabbit and a "back massager," sexual taboos were continuously tackled and broken down. Lots of women watched every Sunday night, and the show gave them permission to talk about sexual feeling (and sexual healing) around the water cooler, in restaurants, or in the bedroom. *Sex and the City*, with its dynamic, frank, funny, and sometimes controversial stance on doing it, left a permanent mark on how society views female sexuality.

And yet none of this meant that society was actually ready to see a woman in action. Britain's Channel 4 found that out during an episode of its version of the reality show *Big Brother*. The 2005 cast members discovered one of their housemates, a woman called Kinga, pleasuring herself with an empty wine bottle in an episode that aired to six million U.K. viewers. Calls flooded in complaining about the direction of the show. And yet, through the fallout, it was clear that the episode received a lot more attention because it was a woman, not a guy, masturbating on TV. As Lebby Eyres wrote in *Bint* magazine, "While Kinga's behavior was, erm, surprising, and not very sensible, it seems it was the fact that female masturbation was involved that most shocked the viewers."[15]

In July 2006, Channel 4 was at it again. This time its plan was to broadcast London's version of the San Francisco Masturbate-a-thon. Lester Haines, a journalist with the *Register* in the United Kingdom, likened masturbation to porn, and went on to share his disgust around the event, calling the Masturbate-a-thon a piece of U.S. "degeneracy." On the flip side, indie production company Zig Zag, which was scheduled to film the event, said in a press release: "This year it's time to bring the event across the pond to see if the great British public can embrace mass public masturbation. It's time to find out if the only things allowed to be stiff in Britain are upper lips."[16] Channel 4 ultimately pulled its decision to air London's Masturbate-a-thon, citing the fallout from *Big Brother* as its reason.[17]

> *"I think masturbation is a lot more accepted than it ever was before. Sex stores and books have become more prevalent, and I do believe that men enjoy women's newfound masturbation freedom."*
>
> —Ilene, age twenty-six

With all the controversy around masturbation on television, it's important to see things as they still are. While rape and murder are freely broadcast at all hours of the day on the news and on popular TV shows, female sexuality and masturbation are still regarded as heavy-hitting, hard-to-digest subjects. Is it that coming into our own personal power through sexuality is scarier than somebody else exerting power over us? I know the answer's no, but television doesn't seem to agree.

## MASTURBATION in BLACK-and-WHITE

Everyone has a favorite when it comes to silver-screen sex scenes. For me the most beautiful depiction of female masturbation in film can be found in the 1998 movie *Pleasantville*. Here, two teenagers are transported into their television set, only to find themselves living in a black-and-white TV-town called Pleasantville, where everything is as innocent as *Leave It to Beaver*. When the sexually repressed mom, Betty Parker (Joan Allen), asks her daughter, Mary Sue (Reese Witherspoon), what goes on at the local hangout Lovers Lane, Mary Sue tells her that sex goes on there. This leaves Betty to probe further: "What's sex?" Mary Sue proceeds to explain the birds and the bees to her mother. Betty tells Mary Sue that her father would never do that, and Mary Sue tells her mom that there are other ways to enjoy herself without having to involve Dad. The camera pans to a disbelieving yet hopeful Betty, whom we then see turning on the bathtub faucets while her husband goes to sleep in one of their two twin beds.

Inside the bathroom, Betty stands in front of a mirror and strips naked, looking at her body for what appears to be the first time. She then slides into the bath and we hear the rustling of water while Betty figures out where she wants to be touched. As she begins to exclaim, "Oh my goodness!" louder and louder, everything in the black-and-white bathroom—the wallpaper, the bath soaps, the bath salts—starts to bloom with color. The viewer is then taken to the outside of the Parkers' home to the black-and-white image of their front yard, where we are treated to the visual of a tree bursting into bright orange flames at the very same moment that she peaks. To me it symbolizes the mythic power, and fear, of a female orgasm.

> *"I think society's views on masturbation have (at least in metro areas) done a 360. I can see this particularly through my own mother's experiences. She never masturbated and thought it was dirty until five years ago. After she went through a divorce, her therapist suggested masturbating and buying a dildo. Just seeing how much she has changed from this experience—going from a woman who viewed sex as not incredibly pleasurable to a woman who knows what makes her tick and really enjoys sex—it's been amazing to watch."*
>
> *—Alissa, age twenty-five*

 **PRINTED PLEASURES**

Mainstream girlie magazines like *Glamour* and *Cosmo* are more likely to tout the benefits of sex with an ex than sex with yourself. Sure, they'll devote an article every so often to solo pleasure, or they'll throw in a section on sex toys, but most of the writing on the wall is all about finding the perfect male mate. Maybe it's because sex sells better when it's about girl getting guy, or maybe it's because you can sell more products for attracting a mate than you can for becoming attractive to yourself, but the truth is, there's still a ways to go until we truly accept, and embrace, masturbation.

Magazines are happy to spout out the same five sex tips that will make you a better lover, help you land the dude of your dreams, or make your orgasm louder and longer, but they rarely touch on same-sex love or self-pleasure, and they hardly ever call it masturbation. In the April 2007 *Redbook* article "14 Secrets to Feeling Sexier," the magazine advises readers to "toy with self-pleasure." It's a positive single paragraph about masturbation with a sex toy—though actually, it's more about the author using a sex toy and eventually showing her husband how she does it (he previously wasn't interested in toys), which turns both of them on.

Some women get their sex information from more explicit magazines. In fact, lots of women flip through sex magazines like *Penthouse, Playboy,* and *Playgirl*. These magazines allow women to explore their own sexuality through detailed letters, articles, and advice, while providing them with visual "turn-on" stimulation.

> *"Most women's magazines have gotten very detailed, but it's all "how-to": how to have a better orgasm, get him off quicker, be a better lover. Rarely are we allowed to talk about how we feel about sex, how it makes us feel. I think a great thing is that almost every woman I know admits to masturbating. And women have made some great strides in taking responsibility for their own orgasms. I've had many lovers and none of them were the slightest bit surprised when I got on top of them and started touching myself while fucking. I guess that meant I wasn't the only one doing it!"*
>
> —*Christen, age thirty-five*

 **GETTING OFF ONLINE**

The Internet has allowed people to open up and explore masturbation in private, from the comfort of their own couches, beds, and desks. Those of us fortunate enough to have Internet access can find lots of educational, informational, and titillational material online. The Internet makes us feel less alone, and allows us to explore parts of ourselves we'd otherwise never have the opportunity to understand. Today, if you think you have a problem because you masturbate often, or because you don't orgasm from vaginal penetration, you're just a click away from learning that you're one of many women who feel the same way. Years ago, it was absolutely more difficult to have these types of discussions, or to get positive information about female sexuality. Online you can enter a chat room and talk with a complete stranger about anything. You can peruse websites and join in discussions on solo sex, or read about how other women your age feel about their own sexuality. You can find resources, download videos, and read blogs to get both personal and professional perspectives on the subject. Yes, there's a lot of negative messaging about self-sexuality out there still, and yes, some of it's subliminally negative, like when someone "confesses" to masturbation, as if it's a sin, or when someone else uses masturbation to "get back" at her partner for not being a more caring lover, but the Internet is also the most valuable resource around for the mass distribution of positive sexuality information. It reaches beyond the national scope and allows us to communicate universally with other women, allowing those who can access the Internet the chance to both educate and get an education.

Aside from knowledge, the Internet provides us with oodles and oodles of fodder for getting off. There is an abundance of erotica and pornography available and accessible (and even free) for women to read or view to help them with the task at hand (see Chapter 9: Enticement). Of course, there are also a lot of negative images of sexuality out there, but the more we frequent the places that feed our power, the less those other bad places will affect us. The more we spread the word about positive sexuality, the more positive images of sexuality will be out there for us to view. No matter how you surf it, the Internet is a great way to enjoy masturbation without shame, guilt, or fear. Without it we'd be in a much sadder state of sexual satisfaction, knowledge, and empowerment.

> *"Every now and then I'll look at naked pictures or watch porn. I've found that men enjoy putting pictures of their penises online. Craigslist is a great place to find free penis porn. There are some rather lovely specimens to view. I have to admit, though, that the one thing that has turned me on more than anything is sharing erotic stories and real-time scenarios with lovers via email or IM. It gives me a sense of connection with someone and leaves room for pseudoanonymity. I've gotten so turned on by cybersex with a long-distance lover that I've had a G-spot orgasm while sitting in my chair typing. Damn, that was hot!"*
>
> —Mischa, age thirty-five

## ABSTAINING FROM SEX SHOULD NOT MEAN ABSTAINING FROM MASTURBATION

 **FACT** "The welfare reform legislation signed into law by President Clinton in August of 1996 represents—to date—the broadest attack on the provision of comprehensive sexuality education to young people in the United States."

—Sexuality Information and Education Council of the United States[18]

The United States' current policy on sex education is "abstinence only." Before 1996, the U.S. government abided by the 1919 White House Conference on Child Welfare, which stated that sex education was the schools' responsibility. Now the only type of sex education the federal government will fund for young women and men across the country is the type of education that teaches them to "just say no" to all types of sex. The government sees this as the best way to effectively prevent disease and pregnancy, and therefore spent $176 million in 2007 on promoting its abstinence-only agenda. Research shows that this type of "education" is never discussed honestly. The logic is that young adults who don't have sex don't need to protect themselves, so there's little, if any, talk about condoms, touching, or sexual activity going on in these classrooms. Schools that follow the "abstinence only" guidelines get tax breaks and incentives while continuing to shun the fact that it's human nature to feel and be sexual. Studies, research, and the high rates of pregnancy among unwed teenagers in this country prove that young women are still going to have sex, no matter what they're not taught in schools. So what do schools teach about masturbation, which is, by far, the safest sex out there? Almost as much as they teach about sex. Maybe they tell you masturbation's healthy, but odds are, they don't say a word.

> *"There is not much taught in schools about masturbation, especially for girls or women. I haven't seen any data on what is taught about masturbation or even if it is taught, but from everything I know, it's not. I do know that when I suggest that adults talk about masturbation with young girls because it might be a really good way to help young girls abstain from sex with a partner (if abstinence is indeed what the adults would urge them to practice), the adults are mortified that masturbation is even suggested."*
>
> —*Konnie McCaffree, PhD, AASECT-certified sexuality educator, certified family life educator*

## ONE MODERN MAMA

Not all parents shiver at the thought of their children masturbating. M. B., a thirty-two-year-old modern mother who is both a birth worker and a yoga teacher, has an enlightened approach to her daughter's self-pleasure:

"My daughter has been touching, feeling, and exploring herself from the time she was at least a year old," she says. "She is three and a half now and just recently we have very, very subtly addressed the subject. She likes to do it on the couch while she is watching a movie. We tell her that touching her yoni is fine, fun, and sacred. We don't mind that she does it in the living room while watching a DVD (she doesn't get into it, she just smiles and watches Pooh Bear as her fingers wander in her yoni and rectal area), but if other people are over we tell her she should go into her private bedroom because it is a private act.

"I will let my daughters lead me . . . I will never ever make them feel shamed, obviously, but I also will honor their own personal boundaries and never push them into talking about masturbation. I will gently give them the lowdown bit by bit as they mature, but we will keep it gentle. It is sacred, and it is personal; it's making love to ourselves . . . what a beautiful and empowering act! I want them to feel they have the privacy they deserve without a mother's knowing eye. I also encourage them to explore their bodies in many other ways, like breathing, doing yoga, dancing, tumbling, massage, and energy work. To feel comfortable in this skin, in these temples, truly ensures us a path of spiritual freedom, as well as sexual freedom (they so go hand in hand).

"I hope that masturbation becomes something normal and delicious to both my daughters, and I long for them to have amazing sex lives. I hope that that my girls choose masturbation for many, many years before they choose partners. I say this mainly because if they get to know their own bodies, needs, and desires, they surely will be mature and responsible lovers. I also say this because hopefully through self-exploration they'll find more love for themselves, so when they choose to have sex with another, they choose to because of that deep love they have cultivated within and they long to share that."

## IT'S NOT A NEED, IT'S A WANT

Women don't need to masturbate. For most of us it's not a primal urge, a sudden "must-do" way of releasing the pent-up energy we feel we have to free into the universe. Most women masturbate because they like how it feels, or they want to know what it feels like because maybe they've never had an orgasm before. Women who masturbate are open to the sensations going on in their body. We don't think of masturbation as a reward for being good, or as consolation for being alone. This might surprise you, but more women masturbate when they're having sex or are sexually fulfilled than when they aren't. Masturbation isn't something we have to do, but it's something a lot of us like to do.

These days, women are waiting longer to meet "the one" and to settle down into a routine that involves children and a mortgage. Today's city chick is often more focused on herself and her indulgences, and she is more open to and accepting of the part masturbation plays in her life. Of course, this is a generalization, but I see it in my friends, coworkers, and family. Today's young professional women are more in touch with their own wants and desires, and, rather than trying to fulfill their every sexual satisfaction through the discovery of someone else, they know how to take matters into their own hands.

### BETTY DODSON: SEX ARTIST

She's been called the mother of masturbation, and then the grandmother, and for a while she was even called the godmother of masturbation. It doesn't matter what you call her; if you know anything about "liberating masturbation" and the biggest movement to accept self-sexuality as first-rate sex, then you've heard of Betty Dodson. If not, you'll know her well by the end of this book. Native Americans honor grandmother wisdom, and these are her words.

➡

### IN THE BEGINNING

"I got divorced in 1965, and by 1968 I was going to sex parties and experiencing anything I ever had a fantasy about. It was fabulous! Then I started having my own group sex parties, and it got even better because I could invite the right mix of people—like creating the ideal dinner party. From my group sex experiences I could see that the guys knew what they wanted; they were getting off and having a ball. Meanwhile, far too many women were accommodating the men and faking orgasms. As a budding feminist, I felt this was unacceptable. Women had to learn what they needed and how to get what they wanted in order to enjoy their orgasms. This became my feminist commitment when I began running nude masturbation workshops for women.

"In the early '70s I was a part of the grassroots feminist movement that was based upon consciousness-raising (CR) groups. All we had to do was get a group of women together and share our experiences using "I" statements. These were very powerful gatherings, but they were about everything but sex—salary, housework, paid leave for pregnancy, birth control, abortion—not a word about women's sexual pleasure. In 1972 I started my Bodysex groups, for feminists who wanted to take sex into their own hands. Although I imagined I'd run these groups for a couple of years and then get back to my art, the workshops occupied me for the next twenty-two years.

"At the 1973 NOW conference I ran a workshop that introduced electric vibrators, and on Sunday I showed slides of female genitals to over a thousand women in the main auditorium. Imagine projecting six-foot images of vulvas at the first and last Sex Conference that the National Organization for Women ever held. I produced portraits of fifteen women. Our poses consisted of one natural photo, one with the outer lips held open, one with the clitoral glans exposed, and the last one had each woman arranging her vulva the way she thought it looked

➡

best. As a slide appeared on the screen, I described each one using the word *cunt,* the old Anglo-Saxon noun that goes with *cock.* 'This one is a Danish modern cunt, this next one is an art deco cunt,' and so on. I wanted to reclaim the word, but to this day many women hate the word *cunt.*"

## ON PARTNERS AND G-SPOTS

"When I was married I secretly masturbated while my former husband slept in bed next to me. I didn't get to come very often during partnersex because he came too fast, and it was too difficult for me to get off from fucking only. We were far too inhibited to try other forms of sex. A man and a woman fucking with the guy on top equaled sex, and, while society has made some progress, that's still the most common image of partnersex today. How unlady-like for a woman to reach down to stimulate her clitoris during intercourse! She should be coming from penis/vagina penetration with her monogamous husband, getting pregnant, having babies, and being normal.

"Today there is a resurgence of women who want vaginal orgasms thanks to the G-spot. But the vagina is not our primary sex organ, even though the female sex organ is often called a 'vagina.' While there are some nerve endings at the outer part of the vaginal opening, and some women have vaginal orgasms, most of us prefer some form of direct clitoral stimulation along with vaginal penetration. I think the G-spot has been overstated. Based upon thirty years of working with women, orgasms from G-spot stimulation alone are very inconsistent and not for every woman. Still, people believe that being inside someone's body, from a French kiss to fingering her G-spot, is more passionate than doing her clit. Why not do all of it?

"Unfortunately, the G-spot and female ejaculation have become one more thing that women have to master to be sexually fashionable. Too many people think they're proof that a woman has had an orgasm, but that's not always true. Women can squirt without having one. Before diving

➡

back into the vagina, looking for a 'spot,' I'd encourage women to spend more time getting to know their clitoris, which is a more consistent source of pleasure."

### ON THE STATE OF THE SEXUAL UNION

"We're much more accepting of dirty politics than we are of kinky sex. Anything that deviates from mom-and-pop monogamous marital sex is suspect in middle America. Meanwhile, our corrupt government officials, church leaders, and other men of power ignore this strict Puritan morality as they hire professionals to sexually entertain them, keeping the sexual double standard thriving while they pretend to be faithful or chaste.

"Each new generation has to reinvent the wheel all over again. Until we have decent sex education in the lower grades, sexual ignorance will continue. If kids haven't learned that it's okay to be sexual with themselves by the time they reach high school, their sexual development has been damaged. By blocking comprehensive sex education that honors masturbation, includes sex information, and teaches birth control, we are actually preventing our children from having fulfilling adult sex lives."

### ON MASTURBATION

"Basically, we are born masturbators. Without any prohibition, children will naturally reach down and play with their fascinating sex organ. It's how we discover and learn to like our genitals. Sexual conditioning begins at the nonverbal level with how a mother washes her baby's genitals. I had the good fortune of talking to my mom about the fear that I had been born with a genital deformity—inner lips that dangled. My mother admitted that she thought there might have been something wrong with my baby vulva. Until I was thirty-five, I thought I'd stretched my inner lips from too much childhood masturbation. Finally, my first postmarital lover showed me his 'split beaver' girlie magazines and I realized I was 'normal.' After years of running workshops

➡

where we did Genital Show and Tell, I'd estimate that more than half of the women had beautiful drapery with long inner lips that I named 'Renaissance cunts.'

"There are just so many ways we can be sexual, but it begins with self-sexuality. Once that's in place we can go on to enjoy partnersex, threesomes, foursomes—or five or more (which would be group sex). Or we can be celibate. Or simply self-sexual. Or we can choose to be traditional with a lifetime of monogamous marital sex. One thing is clear: Until society accepts and honors masturbation as the foundation for all of human sexuality, people will continue to be manipulated through sexual shame and guilt by any authoritarian government or religion that comes along."

### ON ORGASM

"I think every woman is capable of having orgasms, even though it's not a requirement to have had one in order to give birth. A man has to ejaculate to impregnate a woman. He's assured of having an orgasm because his climax accompanies ejaculation. If a woman's clitoris were big enough to move in and out of a wet orifice, female orgasm wouldn't be such a mystery. A woman's ability to orgasm is more complex because it depends upon her mental, physical, and emotional state. Being in love is often a woman's favorite aphrodisiac, and then she often doesn't care if she comes. One of the best things about masturbation is knowing that orgasm is a given. In the end, we must remember that there is no such thing as having a 'wrong' kind of orgasm. An orgasm is an orgasm is an orgasm. It's all good."

### ON SEXUAL FANTASY

"The one thing I appreciate more since I've gotten older is sexual fantasy. It's absolutely the best way for me to focus my mind and stop running the grocery list in my head. I've given myself permission to fantasize about anything. I start going through my Rolodex of dirty fantasies, looking for one that sparks my interest. I can begin running one and

> then change to another, put two together, or add something new to a golden oldie. One thing is sure: The thought police are not allowed to interfere with my delicious perversions."
>
> **SEXUALLY SPEAKING, TODAY**
>
> "During the first seven years of my seventies I had some of the hottest orgasmic partnersex of my life. It was totally unexpected. Before I met Eric, I was perfectly willing to be done with heterosexuality. If I was ever going to live with a lover again, I thought it would be a woman. Heterosexuality took me through the same pattern again and again: I'd fall into lust while calling it love, enjoy the first three months or year of hot sex, and then spend the next year or so breaking up. After living happily and sexually with Eric into the ninth year of our relationship, I'm currently going through another transition. Although Eric and I have never been monogamous, I told him I wanted to get more into my own sexuality. This past year I've started to travel more, I'm meditating again, and I'm no longer dependent on partnersex for my best orgasms. It's a good feeling to own myself, to own my body, and to be the creator of my own world. That doesn't mean I won't occasionally take advantage of living with a very handsome young man who is a skilled lover."

 ## CONTINUING EDUCATION

It would be fantastic to say that the current view of masturbation has changed so much from its deeply buried past. The truth is that we do talk about it a little more than we used to, but not as much as we need to. We need to embrace the fact that we can get ourselves off, and that we hold the key to unlocking our own boxes.

Yes, more women are talking about their sexual satisfaction with both partners and friends, and lots more women are open to exploring their sexuality beyond partnersex. Sex stores, and the emergence of the boutique sex shop, have really helped women transition from dependent partners to independent sex-toy consumers and self-pleasurers. Self-help books, celebrity confessions (even sex tapes), and talk show TV have all helped women embrace their sexuality, but for each woman who's one step ahead, there's another woman who needs a helping hand to move forward.

Until we teach comprehensive sexuality education that emphasizes masturbation, and until we teach younger people that touching themselves isn't the equivalent of a late-night horror show, we have a ways to go in improving the sexual culture of our youth. When we emphasize abstinence we neglect to remind ourselves (and others) of the importance of loving our own bodies. Until we tell our daughters, sisters, friends, and lovers that masturbation is sex with someone you love and that it's okay to enjoy self-pleasure, we are not as far along as we need to be in terms of our selfless acceptance of self-love.

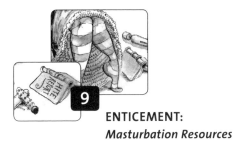

## 9

### ENTICEMENT:
### *Masturbation Resources*

WHETHER YOU USE YOUR MIND, your Mac, or magazines, there are lots of resources that can aid you in your quest for masturbation material. Below are links to a sampling of them.

## REQUIRED READING

It would be great if our bodies came with instruction manuals, but since they don't we have to learn what we know on our own. The following books offer information on our bodies and our sexual health. Not only are most of them jam-packed with information, they're also great to share among friends.

### GRRL POWER: REQUIRED READING ON POLITICS, SEX, AND OUR BODIES

*The Clitoral Truth: The Secret World at Your Fingertips,* by Rebecca Chalker (Seven Stories Press, 2000)

> This is seriously the best book ever on the clitoris! It's got everything you'd need or want to know about your best bud and it's a totally easy read, with even easier to understand diagrams and illustrations.

*Femalia,* edited by Joani Blank (Down There Press, 1993)

>An entire book of photography dedicated to images of women's genitals; there is a whole variety of shapes, sizes, and colors represented here. A fantastic book to help women realize how many different vulvas exist and how exquisitely detailed each one is.

*For Yourself: The Fulfillment of Female Sexuality,* by Lonnie Barbach (Signet, revised 2000)

>This book, written by a sex therapist, offers a step-by-step program allowing women to better understand and be comfortable with their own sexuality. With lots of clear, factual advice that's presented in simple language and a style that's warm and positive, it's got effective exercises to help women fulfill their sexual potential.

*The Good Vibrations Guide: The G-Spot,* by Cathy Winks (Down There Press, 1998)

>If you want more information on how your body works, this book, which is more the size of a pamphlet than a novel, will provide you with the basics you need to know about what the G-spot is—and how to find it.

*The G-Spot: And Other Discoveries About Human Sexuality,* by Beverly Whipple, John D. Perry, and Alice Kahn Ladas (Owl Books, reprinted 2004)

>If you want even more detail on the G-spot, this book will provide you with what you're looking for. Some of the research is a little outdated, and it's not the most exciting read, but it was the first book of its kind on the subject. It was *the* book to conclude that the G-spot did, in fact, exist.

**A New View of a Woman's Body, by the Federation of Feminist Women's Health Centers (Feminist Health Press, 1995)**

This book is filled with lots of medical and technical jargon about women's bodies, but that's because the Federation spent years teaching women how to fend for themselves. It's the book responsible for redefining the clitoris, and it includes chapters on how to take responsibility for your own maintenance and upkeep (in the form of things like self-breast and vaginal/cervical exams). It's also got a great chapter on birth control and another section on feminist abortion care. Not a book about masturbation—in fact, there's not much on the subject—but a book that every woman should own in order to better understand the mechanics of her body.

**Our Bodies, Ourselves: A New Edition for a New Era, by the Boston Women's Health Book Collective (Touchstone, 2005)**

Again not a book on masturbation, but a book that details the social, cultural, and psychological effects of growing up female. Addressing issues from body image to sexuality to political reform, this book is an essential read for women who care not only about their bodies, but also about the state of being female. A sociocultural cult favorite— your mother may even have a copy of the original on her bookshelf.

**The Science of Orgasm, by Barry R. Komisaruk, Carlos Beyer-Flores, and Beverly Whipple (Johns Hopkins University Press, 2006)**

If you're the kind of girl who likes to know everything you can about how your body works, then this book on orgasms is definitely one-of-a-kind research. A neuroscientist, an endocrinologist, and a sex researcher delve into the connection between the brain and the genitals and come to the conclusion that the brain is indeed the most powerful sex organ.

*Sex for One: The Joy of Selfloving,* by Betty Dodson (Three Rivers Press, reissued 1996)

Dodson's personal journey from small-town Kansas girl to grand-mother of masturbation is not only inspirational, but informational. Dodson is more than just funny and opinionated; she's a talented writer and fine artist. Her insight into self-love, and sexuality in general, makes this a quick read.

*The Smart Girl's Guide to the G-Spot,* by Violet Blue (Cleis Press, 2007)

If you're looking for a book with more than the G-spot basics, check out Violet Blue's book on the subject. This book includes advanced positions, techniques, and information on ejaculation. Plus, erotic writer Alison Tyler adds extra oomph with her steamy stories.

## MASTURBATION FROM A HISTORICAL PERSPECTIVE

Sometimes too much researched reading—the type that has lots of footnotes, endnotes, and citations—needs to be digested in small bites and swallows. But even if it takes you some time to chew through these, they are some of the most interesting books on the subject of masturbation that you'll ever bite into.

*The Big Book of Masturbation,* by Martha Cornog (Down There Press, 2003)

This book covers self-love from angst to zeal, and it looks at masturbation from a variety of perspectives. It even includes a section on how other animals do it. It's a thoughtful and smart look at all the brouhaha that surrounds the subject at hand.

*Solitary Sex: A Cultural History of Masturbation,* by Thomas W. Laqueur
(Zone Books, 2003)

> For the history buff, this is the most comprehensive history of mastur-
> bation anywhere! You'll be able to wow anyone with all this informa-
> tion, and you'll sound so smart in doing so. It's well written, even if it
> feels a bit long at times, but maybe that's because it's so thorough.

*The Technology of Orgasm: "Hysteria," the Vibrator, and Women's Sexual
Satisfaction,* by Rachel P. Maines (Johns Hopkins University Press, 1998)

> If you've ever had a fascination with vibration, this book will tell you
> everything you ever needed to know about the origins of the buzz.
> Maines provides a detailed history of the vibe, and what you learn
> might shock you, but not in the way that your plug-in vibe would if
> you used it in the bathtub.

## FANTASY

Books on fantasy can vary from the instructional to the turn-on-able. Since
you can find links to authors who write erotica in the "Sex-Positive People
and Places" section, this section is small, and includes books that not only
provide fodder for masturbation, but deconstruct our fantasies as well.

*The Erotic Mind: Unlocking the Inner Sources of Passion and Fulfillment,*
by Jack Morin (Harper, reprinted 1996)

> Focusing on our erotic psyches, Morin, along with his three hundred–
> plus respondents, discusses arousal and erotic patterns. This is a
> book that will help you understand your fantasies and enjoy your
> sexual self.

*My Secret Garden,* by Nancy Friday (Pocket Books, 1973)

> This is the groundbreaking book that first looked into women's sexual fantasies. Most of this book is full of detailed fantasies that are easy to get off to, but there's also some insightful commentary provided by the author.

*The Ultimate Guide to Sexual Fantasy: How to Turn Your Fantasies into Reality,* by Violet Blue (Cleis Press, 2004)

> Violet Blue is one of the hottest sex writers around, and her easy-to-read guides are a must-have for any sex-ed library. This one's got a first chapter on fantasy for one, with a section titled "Masturbation: Just Do It." Of course, there are also lots of fantasy ideas for two, but whether you're single or partnered, it doesn't matter—this book is hot. With erotica by Alison Tyler interspersed, it's the complete package.

*Women on Top,* by Nancy Friday (Pocket Books, 1991)

> My favorite of the *My Secret Garden* trilogy, because it's the first (and last) book of Friday's to address masturbation. Friday is easy to read, and has lots to say not only on that subject, but on the subject of mothers and daughters. Plus, after reading the author's commentary, you get to read sexy fantasies written by real women. How hot is that?

## ALL-AROUND-AWESOME SEX BOOKS

If you're looking for a lot of information on a number of topics, check out these excellent picks.

### *The Big Bang: Nerve's Guide to the New Sexual Universe,* by Em and Lo (Plume, 2003)

> Because it was written by sex hipsters Em and Lo, this is probably the coolest-looking sex book around. Really contemporary language, and beautiful, natural, and—you guessed it—hip pictures of hot young model types, grace the pages of this stylish guidebook. I love that the information is delivered in a more conversational manner, and that the book itself is so aesthetically appealing.

### *The Good Vibrations Guide to Sex,* by Cathy Winks and Anne Semans (Cleis Press, 2002)

> Since its first publication in 1994, *The Good Vibrations Guide to Sex* has established itself as a complete and educational sex book. Written by two women who have worked extensively in the sex toy industry, it's a great choice for all your sexual needs.

### *Guide to Getting It On,* by Paul Joannides (Goofy Foot Press, 2006)

> Written by a research psychoanalyst with a sense of humor, the 846 pages of text include a 50-page glossary on every word with any sort of sexual connotation, from *aardvarking* to *yohimbine.* Editions are updated with more regularity than any other sex book. Probably the one sex book to own if you own only one sex book.

*Nina Hartley's Guide to Total Sex,* by Nina Hartley with I. S. Levine
(Penguin, 2006)

> A book about sex by a woman who's been having it, on- and offscreen, for twenty-five years. Nina Hartley is the perfect adult performer, sex activist, and educator to pen a total sex book. Her advice is personal and professional, and I love that her experience lets her share so many firsthand accounts.

*Sex with the Lights On,* by Ducky Doolittle (Carroll & Graf, 2006)

> Ducky is a sex educator, writer and witty lady, and that makes for a nice mix when it comes to talking sex. Here she answers 200 "illuminating" sex questions. Reading Ducky is like getting advice from a best girlfriend. The book is full of honest, positive and affirming sex advice, and it's all easy to digest!

 **TOYING WITH MASTURBATION**

The following is a list of many of the toys mentioned earlier in this book, plus a few books that are worth reading if you want to learn more about sex toys. These are the types of toys you didn't get to play with as a child.

### GUIDES TO VIBRATORS AND OTHER SEX TOYS

If you want even more information on vibes and/or other sex toys, you can check out any of the following fantastic resources:

*The Adventurous Couple's Guide to Sex Toys,* by Violet Blue
(Cleis Press, 2006)

> This fun and well-researched consumer guide to sex toys will allow you to further explore anything you need to know on the subject. Plus,

Ms. Blue offers some interesting ideas on how to incorporate toys into your relationship.

### *Em and Lo's Sex Toys: An A–Z Guide to Bedside Accessories,* by Em and Lo (Chronicle Books, 2006)

One of the most comprehensive guides, it starts at A and ends at Z. Fun, honest, and easy to read, this is a great accessory for anyone who uses, or wants to use, sex toys.

### *Good Vibrations: The New Complete Guide to Vibrators,* by Joani Blank and Ann Whidden (Down There Press, 2000)

It's slim, but that doesn't mean it's not power-packed with information on all things vibrating. If you're looking to buy your first vibe, or your second, this book can help. Unfortunately, it hasn't been updated since 2000, but it's got lots of personal anecdotes and stories from some of the women responsible for bringing vibrators to a larger, more mainstream market.

### *Sex Toys 101: A Playfully Uninhibited Guide,* by Rachel Venning and Claire Cavanah (Fireside, 2003)

The bright, beautiful pictures make this book easy on the eyes. Although some toys in this guide have died and gone to sex toy heaven, the book is still a fantastic introduction to the great wide world of sex toys. The authors, who both happen to be the owners of the world-famous sex shop Babeland, share personal anecdotes and offer advice throughout the book as well. The most picturesque book on sex toys, it's a really pretty read.

## THINGS THAT GO *BUZZ* IN THE NIGHT

The following is a list of sites that are known for manufacturing/selling vibrating toys. Of course, some sites sell lots of other things (like condoms, dildos, and blindfolds), and some don't sell anything at all, but regardless, if you're looking to buy, or just for research, these are places you should know about.

### Durex
### www.durex.com

Durex not only makes sex toys, it makes lubes and condoms as well. The lubes and condoms are often available at the same places you'd purchase your toilet paper and other household supplies from, but you can't find Durex's five years of global sex surveys or their vibrators in drugstores. So check out their online home for all that jazz.

### Funfactory
### www.funfactory.de

Funfactory doesn't actually have walk-in stores, but if you want a closer look at its line of silicone vibes, Smartballs, and anal toys you can check out its virtual showroom and then head to an online retailer to find the silicone vibe or butt toy of your dreams.

### Natural Contours
### www.natural-contours.com

Ergonomically engineered to fit the curves of a woman's body, the Natural Contours line of hard plastic vibes includes the Ultime and the Idéal. Leading the market in cool, unique designs, it also has a lot of other beautiful vibes to check out, especially the Jolie and the Liberté.

## OhMiBod
## www.ohmibod.com

If you're the kind of girl who is always connected to her MP3 player or cell phone, then this is the site—and product—for you. The original OhMiBod hooks up to your favorite MP3 player, and its newest vibe, Boditalk, is activated by calls to or from your cell phone. You can join Club Vibe, get more information, and buy their products online on this site.

## Rocks-Off Limited
## www.rock-chick.com

The Rock-Chick is the first toy to come from the company Rocks-Off Limited, and its great curved design can literally rock your world. You can buy the toy on the site, or you can buy the toy from a site in the United States and save a lot of money on shipping.

## The TriGasm
## www.avacadell.com

This is the link to the home of the triple-action jelly rubber TriGasm, as well as other toys recommended (and sometimes created) by Dr. Ava Cadell, the media therapist and self-proclaimed love guru.

## Vibratex
## www.vibratex.com

This is the site for the company that makes the Water Dancer, the Rabbit Habit, and a lot of the other most popular dual-action vibes. The site isn't a place where you can buy the toys, but you'll find a little information on the materials they use. For purchasing, check out the list of retail stores.

### Wahl

**www.wahl-store.com**

Click the link to Health Care and then follow that to Swedish-Style Massagers, and you'll find the largest offering of Wahl vibrators around. They may not call them the 7-in-1, but they've got all the parts you need for any kind of massage.

### LUXURY SEX

For a more detailed look at the following vibrators, check out chapter 3, "The Buzz."

### Elemental Pleasures

**www.elementalpleasures.com**

Elemental Pleasures' high-end vibrators are the ones made out of aircraft-caliber materials. They're the priciest vibes of the bunch, but if you're all about the highest quality materials, then these might be the vibes for you. You can buy them directly from the site.

### Emotional Bliss

**www.emotionalbliss.com**

The creators of Emotional Bliss's line of somewhat sterile-looking vibrators took five years to come up with the perfect buzz. Each one is designed a tad bit differently, so that women with different needs can find the right one for them. Emotional Bliss vibes are serious about women's sexuality. To buy them in the United States, check out one of the retailers listed later in the chapter.

### Eroscillator

**www.eroscillator.com**

The sensual toy that oscillates instead of vibrates—online you can choose from five different packages, each with different heads. It's quiet, strong, and never needs batteries, and it's my new favorite personal vibrating sex toy. Buy it online from their store; plus, read lots more about the massager on their website.

### Je Joue

**www.jejoue.com**

*Je joue* literally translates to "I play." The Je Joue sensual massager has been created with the idea that foreplay is an important part of more play. It grooves with your body, quivering, swirling and gliding all over your clit, to get you dancing to orgasm. The site's got a cool section called the O Zone, and under Pleasure Principles there's another fun section on solo play. It's a U.K. site, so buying online might be easier if you do it in the United States.

### Jimmyjane

**www.jimmyjane.com**

Jimmyjane's vibes are all about the details, from the materials to the etchings. If you're looking for an everlasting vibrator, not to be confused with the everlasting gobstopper, then you'll find it in their sleek and smart vibes with the only patented replaceable motors. You can buy them online here, too.

### Lelo

**www.lelo.com**

> Lelo's motto is "lust objectified," and they don't cut corners when it comes to style and pleasure. Beautiful, artistic, and hardworking, these rechargeable vibes are all state-of-the-art and from Sweden. You can buy them online, but if you want to save on shipping, search around.

### Twisted Products's Cone

**www.conezone.org**

> The partially penetrative pink pointy pleasure cap of vibration has sixteen fantastic pulsations and vibrations for you to ride along to. Plus, the unique shape allows you to place the Cone on the floor, on the wall, or in between your thighs to get you off any which way you want. The music's a little much on the site, but I love how interactive the site is, and it's fun to play with the virtual Cone. While you can't buy the Cone here, you can find a list of retailers under the Buy the Cone tab on the site.

## DILDOS, BUTT STUFF, AND OTHER TYPES OF TOYS

The following is a list of websites for the products in chapter 4's guide to phthalate-free sex toys. If you don't see a link to the toy you want here, odds are, you can find it online at any of the retailers listed later in the chapter.

### Aneros

**www.aneros.com**

> Even though the page touts itself as the home of the best male G-spot stimulators (and they are), the truth is that Aneros's newest toy doesn't discriminate. All Aneros toys are made of high-grade hard plastic, and the one that's being touted for both sexes is called the

Peridise. You can shop online, where Aneros offers lots of package deals on a number of their goodies.

### Feeldoe
**www.feeldoe.com**

This website is not luxurious, but if you're looking to get down to feel-good business, you've come to the right place. There's additional information on the product, and you can shop here! (Purchase any of the six available feeldoes—three colors, all with or without vibration.) Plus, learn more about their other hot toy, the Acrylic Transfer.

### The Massage Stone
**www.themassagestone.com**

The Massage Stone's motto is, "Designed to aid the hands, not replace them," and while there are lots of uses for these stones, they do make for great sex toys. You can heat them and chill them, and they're obviously sturdy (they're stone). Buy them online here.

### njoy
**www.njoytoys.com**

Home of the most beautiful stainless steel toys, njoy is total luxury for your pussy or bum. You can't buy toys directly from the site, but they'll let you know where you can pick up their Pure Wand, their Fun Wand, or any one of their three sizes of butt plugs.

### Phallix
**www.phallixglass.com**

Over four hundred glass artisans make Phallix glass toys. Phallix toys are 100 percent handblown, functional pieces of erotic art. Made from high-quality, medical-grade Pyrex glass, they are hypoallergenic and safe, and can even be thrown in the dishwasher. Plus, the toys don't fade and the colors won't bleed. These glass toys are the kind of toys you can keep on the coffee table, and you can shop online and choose from a multitude of styles and colors.

**Tantus**

**www.tantusinc.com**

Tantus silicone toys are safe, pleasurable, and 100 percent silicone. Each toy is generally available in three colors, and some come with vibration. The newest line is the Dual Density 02 line, which is softer than your garden-variety silicone. If you click on the Find a Retailer link (under Where to Buy), you'll be hooked up with Tantus Direct, your one-stop shop for all your Tantus silicone needs.

**Vixen Creations**

**www.vixencreations.com**

Vixen has been making quality silicone dildos and butt plugs since 1992. Their products are handcrafted and come with a lifetime guarantee. Their VixSkin material is super close to the real deal and other of their silicone toys come in colors that shimmer. You can check out their best-sellers, get handy tips about choosing your new pleasure buddy, and order online here too.

**Xhale Glass**

**www.xhaleglass.com**

I love that Xhale makes a glass toy with hearts, but it's only one of the company's many options. Like Phallix's, their toys aren't only aesthetically appealing but feel really nice inside of you. From twenty-four-carat gold to abstract works of art, you can find yourself a nice glass toy here, and order online.

## Waterpik
### www.waterpik.com

If you're looking for shower power to help you in your masturbatory endeavors, the fine folks at Waterpik have been leaders in the biz since 1962. You can find more showerheads than you've ever dreamed possible on their website; plus, they'll help you locate a place to purchase the perfect pik to help fulfill your wettest dreams.

## LOVELY LUBES

Not all lubes have their own websites, but the ones that do are listed below. Still, you can usually find them all online at one of the many sex shops I've mentioned in this chapter.

## Astroglide
### www.astroglide.com

Astroglide now makes a glycerin- and paraben-free lube, but it's not the good, old-fashioned glycerin lube the company's famous for. Outside of K-Y, this is the most recognizable lube around. You can get free samples online, as well as learn a little about safer sex and other things in their health and information center.

## Emerita
### www.emerita.com

This is a small woman-owned operation out of Portland, Oregon, that sells wellness products designed for women's health and beauty. You can buy their lubes and other products directly from the site, and you can also check out the Emerita blog while you're there.

### Good Clean Love
**www.goodcleanlove.com**

> Another site with a blog (and a podcast), this is a place where you can also share your own self-love story. The woman behind Good Clean Love is helping women make love sustainable with the most natural lubes, oils, and candles around. Plus, every time you make a purchase, Good Clean Love contributes to the Global Fund for Women, the Breast Cancer Fund's Campaign for Safe Cosmetics, and the Children's Peace Academy.

### ID Lubricants
**www.idlube.com**

> This is a site for information on ID's water-based and silicone lubes, and a place where you can request a free sample. It will also give you links to places where you can purchase the lubes, and you can click on Educational if you want to know more about why you should use lube.

### Liquid Silk and Maximus
**www.liquidsilk.com**

> Bodywise Limited is the manufacturer of two of the lube industry darlings, Liquid Silk and Maximus. The website quotes prices from the United Kingdom, and you can shop online—even though you'll probably find better prices if you buy these lubes somewhere in the United States. You can also learn the latest in Liquid Silk news and learn new words like *androstenol*.

## O'My

### www.omyonline.com

If you want to find out how to use any of the O'My products (which include massage oils, lubes, soy candles, and toys), you can click on a product and learn more about it; you can also find out where to buy it, and whether other people like it. Plus, you can meet the O'My community and learn more about this women-run company.

## Pjur Eros

### www.pjurusa.com

Pjur Eros makes the most popular brand of silicone lube, as well as a host of other fabulous varieties. You can learn all about their different varieties on the site, as well as check out their monthly special offers.

## Probe

### www.davryan.com

The site's not really worth going to unless you want to find a list of online places you can buy Probe. If you're a thorough researcher, then the FAQ section will answer all of your questions about Probe, but there are no free samples offered here.

## Sliquid

### www.sliquid.com

You can't buy any of their glycerin- and paraben-free lubes on their site, but you can buy trucker hats and tanks that boast the brand name. You can find a list of online stores and retail locations, plus learn about all of the Sliquid products at their site.

### Wet
**www.wetinternational.com**

> There's a large FAQ section about why people use Wet products, and if you want to know if Wet uses animal by-products (it doesn't) and which lubes to use where, the site will give you that information. Plus, you can request free samples during specific business hours.

 ## SEX TOYS, GET YOUR SEX TOYS!

A list of places you can shop at to fulfill all your dildo wishes and vibrating dreams.

### Adam and Eve
**www.adameve.com**

> Even though not every product they sell is top of the line, the man behind Adam and Eve, Mr. Phil Harvey, definitely is. Harvey's gone in front of the Supreme Court to defend consumers' right to buy sex toys. According to the company's website, more than 25 percent of Adam and Eve's profits goes toward funding family planning and HIV/AIDS prevention all over the world. Their mail-order catalog is the most popular thing they've got going, but the website has a large selection of (mostly) inexpensive sex toys. Make sure you're okay with their limited privacy policy before you make a purchase.

### Babeland
**www.babeland.com**

> Because I worked at Babeland's New York City stores for over five years, I have more than a small affection for this place. The stores and the website are great, and if you can't make it to one of their four tangible locations (in New York, Seattle, and Los Angeles), you can always shop

online. When you buy from here, know that you're getting great, store-tested, quality products. From anal toys to vibrators, Babeland's got the goods.

## Blowfish
### www.blowfish.com

This site does great product reviews to help you find the best masturbation tool for your shed. Not only are the reviews honest and fun, but they'll tell you what's cool and what's new, and you can even listen to the Radio Blowfish Variety Show podcast to find out more about what's going on in the wonderful world of sex.

## Booty Parlor
### www.bootyparlor.com

My personal favorite part of this site is BP TV. Click on any of Booty Parlor's toys, love kits, body treats, or bedroom accessories, and you'll be able to watch Dana talk you through how to use any of the products. There are no graphic discussions, and, since most sex toys don't come with instructions, Dana is happy to help.

## Come as You Are
### www.comeasyouare.com

Canada's cooperatively run sex toy, book, and video store has a positive, open, fun, and respectful approach to sexuality. If you're in the Toronto area, they also teach workshops and exhibit art at their terrestrial store. If not, you can still check them out on the Internet.

### Early to Bed
### www.early2bed.com

> If you can't make it to the Chicago store, then you can shop Early to Bed online. It's another one of the high-ranking women-oriented, but friendly-to-everyone, types of places.

### EdenFantasys
### www.edenfantasys.com

> This site sells lots of sex toys, but my favorite thing about the site is its sex guides and tips (scroll down to the bottom of the page to find them). The materials guide is super thorough and covers all the bases when it comes to sex toy materials.

### Eros Boutique
### www.erosboutique.com

> Madonna shopped here for a *W* magazine photo shoot because she liked the large selection of equestrian fetish gear. Whatever your fetish or fantasy, Eros Boutique probably has the props you need to make it happen. If you're in the Boston area, you can just drop on in; from anywhere else, order online.

### Eve's Garden
### www.evesgarden.com

> The New York store that's responsible for the first catalog ever catering to women. Founder Dell Williams believed that orgasmic women could save the world, and so in 1974 she set out on her mission to create a place where women's sexuality could grow. If that's not reason enough to visit, I don't know what is.

**Freddy and Eddy**

**www.freddyandeddy.com**

> This is one of the best websites for sex toy reviews, done by a real-life, totally in love couple. They try out every single toy before they sell it! If you're in the Los Angeles area you can stop by their super-cool terrestrial shop, where you're guaranteed to feel like you've just entered their home. If not, join them online.

**Good for Her**

**www.goodforher.com**

> This Canadian-based sex-positive shop hosts the annual Feminist Porn Awards, which acknowledges the people making woman-friendly porn. If you're in Toronto, you can shop in person (and twice a week they offer women/trans-only hours). Otherwise, peruse their shop online.

**Good Vibrations**

**www.goodvibes.com**

> Good Vibrations helped pave the way for most of the sex-positive, noncreepy shops on the list, and they remain at the top of their game. They've got a quality line of their own GV toys and lots of other things to choose from, as well as a GV online zine and GV TV.

**JT's Stockroom**

**www.stockroom.com**

> Yeah, you can get your ball gags, nipple clamps, and floggers at other sex shops, but this is the place to go when you want to really get down with your bad self. It's the oldest adult toy retailer specializing in top-grade bondage gear and fetish wear (in case you also want to dress up for your bad self).

### Purple Passion

**www.purplepassion.com**

If kink is your pleasure, then Purple Passion is another option for shopping. This New York City–based sex shop carries everything from BD/SM toys to medical items, so shop away!

### Smitten Kitten

**www.smittenkittenonline.com**

Like Babeland, Good Vibrations, and Come as You Are, Smitten Kitten hosts a whole line of workshops in its Minneapolis store location. Another of the progressive, superior sex shops in the bunch, Smitten Kitten has the best products on the market, as well as hard-to-find and handcrafted delights.

### A Woman's Touch

**www.a-womans-touch.com**

The kind of place you can feel good about shopping at, this online space calls itself a sexuality resource center, and it is. Owned and operated by a female physician and a female sex educator/counselor, this two-woman operation provides helpful and accurate sex information (including some step-by-step guides), as well as relationship advice. All their products are tested and they only sell safe, effective toys (even though *effective* is subjective). They're committed to carrying as many "green" sex toys as possible, they have a whole vegan product section, and they don't sell any phthalate-laden jelly rubber toys. Plus, there's total privacy and discretion when you place an order. If you're in Wisconsin, check out their two terrestrial shops as well.

### Womyns'Ware

**www.womynsware.com**

> You can download their sex toy guide online and get over one hundred pages of information on a whole lot of sex toys. Dedicated to the celebration of women's sexuality, this consumer advocacy–focused, Vancouver-based shop is all about free trade, and they have a strong focus on doing good. They even feature an exposé section on certain toy manufacturers and what Womyns'Ware considers bad products. This is a fantastic sex shop for the empowered consumer.

 **FEED YOUR MIND**

These online places are good for visual stimulation in either video, auditory, or literary form. For even more titillation, check out the sex-positive people and places listed later in this chapter, where you'll find other great links to material, videos, and resources.

### Abby Winters

**www.abbywinters.com**

> Abby Winters is an erotic site featuring amateur Australian girls. Yes, it's mainly a pay site, but if watching other women masturbate or get it on rings your bell, consider this the jackpot. Every week the site adds two new hours of video and approximately 1,700 new images. One of the most watched sections, Intimate Moments, leaves models alone with a video camera to masturbate. All the stuff on this site is real, which is a large part of the appeal.

### Anna Span's Diary
### www.annaspansdiary.com

Anna Span was Britain's first female porn director, and her production company, Easy on the Eye, produces other people's work as well. I like her stuff because the acting is good (when there is acting), and the actors are real, hot, and fun to watch. Anna is also a member of Feminists Against Censorship, and you can find a list of her films and her stars on her site.

### Beautiful Agony
### www.beautifulagony.com

You don't need to have a subscription to the site to get a taste of what's going on here, but you will get more for your money. It's a site where you watch people getting off from the neck up, so obviously masturbation plays a large role here. (Of course, some of them may be getting fucked by someone else and you'd never know.) Regardless, watch the beautiful faces that lead up to and beyond *la petite mort,* and you'll be inspired to see yourself coming.

### Burning Angel
### www.burningangel.com

Joanna Angel is the founder of the alt porn website dedicated to the celebration of rock 'n' roll, erotic photos, hardcore XXX movies, interviews, and writing. Even though you can see lots more of Joanna Angel in her Burning Angel DVDs, she considers herself a writer first, and you can keep up with her life on the Burning Angel blog. Or you can simply use the site as a reference for some hot alt porn.

## Clean Sheets

### www.cleansheets.com

Fiction, poetry, photos, art, and commentary are all available online at Clean Sheets. Featuring the writing of pros and amateurs, not all of it's good, but you'll be able to find what turns you on. There's a strong sense of community on this site, and that's because since 1998 Clean Sheets has been a destination for anyone who likes literary erotica. New stories are posted weekly.

## Comstock Films

### www.comstockfilms.com

If masturbating to a couple having sex is your thing, it doesn't get any more real than Comstock Films, whose motto is, "Real people, real life, real sex." Each of Tony Comstock's videos is a journey into the intimate lives and love of a real couple. His award-winning erotic documentary films celebrate the sexual intimacy in good relationships. You can buy all his videos here.

## Erotic Readers and Writers Association

### www.erotica-readers.com

This is a site for all readers and writers of erotica. If you're inspired to write, check out their call for submissions. If reading is fundamental, there are two galleries of original erotic fiction for your viewing pleasure, as well as a list of adult movies and information on the latest erotica books. A great place to start or finish your search.

## For the Girls

### www.forthegirls.com

For the Girls is a pay site, and for a monthly charge of twenty-something dollars you can see movies and photos handpicked by women, for women. Plus, get sex advice, tips, a daily blog, reviews, and juicy stories that will help put you in the mood for self-love.

### *Handyman* Video Series
### www.lexingtonsteele.com

This website is the home of the company that makes the Tina Tyler–directed *Handyman* masturbation video series, featuring an assortment of sexy men of all different shapes, colors, and personalities. They all have one thing in common—they're masturbating for the camera. Extremely intimate, at least three volumes are out now, with more to come!

### Hot Movies for Her
### www.hotmoviesforher.com

While this site is great for its blog, sex tips, and interviews with porn's hottest movers and shakers, it's also a great site for watching adult movies. They give you more bang for your buck by offering over seventy thousand titles for download on demand, and you can check out the adult-movie reviews before you purchase. It's got detailed search options, and it's a site written by and for women. Yay!

### I Feel Myself
### www.ifeelmyself.com

From the same folks who bring you Beautiful Agony and Abby Winters, this site is dedicated to ordinary women sharing their orgasms in various stages of undress. You can find all types of erotic titillation here, from interviews and insights to high levels of nudity and sex. Make sure to view the intro movie under the IFM principle on the left-hand side of the screen. It's a pay site, but it's all girls, all the time, and you can contribute too, if you'd like.

## Kara's Erotica for Women
### www.karaslinks.com

Kara's is a place that offers erotica for women, featuring only what the site calls "the best" free erotica (in both written and visual form). You can find lots of goodness here: erotic stories, articles, porn, and links, all available in that one-stop-shopping sort of way, thanks to Kara's links.

## Kink.com
### www.kink.com

If consensual BD/SM is your thing, this San Francisco–based company is where it's at. They pride themselves on the authentic reproduction of genuine BD/SM acts done by and to real people who love to play. If you're into kink, you'll find that this is the place to lead you in the right direction.

## Literotica
### www.literotica.com

Literotica is another one-stop shop for all-original fiction and fantasy sex stories. There's a bulletin board, a live chat, and a weekly advice column—all free on the site.

## Lust Films
### www.lustfilms.com

Lust Films is the brainchild of Erika Lust, a woman with a bachelor's degree in political science focusing on feminism and sociology. Her videos incorporate fresh talent and style.

**Nerve**

**www.nerve.com**

> A smart magazine about sex created for both genders but, as *Nerve* says, created especially for women. Fantastic photography, erotica, and features, as well as blogs, video, and cultural and current events. A good place to go for stimuli and sex news.

**Playgirl**

**www.playgirltv.com**

> Even if you opt out of purchasing Playgirl TV (which has both masturbation scenes and scenes of couples), you can get your daily fix by checking out Playgirl's Hot Bod of the Day. You can also listen to my SexPod podcasts for free (under About Playgirl), and subscribe to the magazine, which not only offers a wide range of naked men, but has sex advice, articles, and original erotica written by and for women.

**Pretty Things Press**

**www.prettythingspress.com**

> From the erotic mind of author, editor, and publisher Alison Tyler comes Pretty Things Press, an imprint dedicated to making erotic fantasies acceptable and available. With titles like *Juicy Erotica*, *Naughty Spanking Stories from A–Z*, and *Down and Dirty*, every girl will be able to find her own masturbation material. You can read a sample of any title before you buy.

**Red Handed Porn**

**www.redhandedporn.com**

> These are the masturbation alternaporn people, and their site is definitely one of the only places to see real people, from all sexual walks of life, feeling the self-love. They are a dyke-owned site, featuring six

new episodes a month, and, while you can browse the site for free, membership has its privileges.

### Scarlet Letters
### www.scarletletters.com

Since 1998 Scarlet Letters has been one of the premiere sites for inspired, intelligent and sex-positive art. From the visual to the written, you can peruse years worth of sexual content that will both arouse and educate.

### Sounds Publishing, Inc.
### www.soundserotic.com

If you're looking for a little audio stimulation next time you masturbate, you can download a steamy tale from Sounds Erotic. You can also purchase CDs of their sugar (tamest), spice (less tame), and spank! (even less tame) stories.

 ## EVEN MORE SEX-POSITIVE PEOPLE AND PLACES ONLINE

### About.com: Sexuality
### www.sexuality.about.com

Cory Silverberg, About.com's guide to sexuality, is one smart cookie. His posts are honest, informative, insightful, and always worth reading. You'll never tire of perusing his archives, and he's got some great stuff on masturbation, lubes, and sex toys.

### Adult DVD Talk—Smart Girls' Porn Reviews
### www.adultdvdtalk.com/reviews/smartgirls.asp

Sex educator Violet Blue created the Smart Girls' Porn Club (you can join at girlpornclub.tribe.net) to allow women a forum for talking about the explicit sexual imagery we enjoy. Adult DVD Talk has given the women of that forum a larger space in which to actually review some of this adult material. Check out their picks and join their club. Oh, and pick up Violet Blue's *The Smart Girl's Guide to Porn* (Cleis Press, 2006) for lots of other great porn info.

### All About My Vagina
### www.myvag.net

The title of this site says it all. With information on masturbation, how to pee standing, DIY sex education, and basically anything else you want to know about being female and sexual, All About My Vagina deserves a look. Sarah from Vancouver runs this site, and, although we've never spoken, her site speaks volumes about how cool she is.

### Annie Sprinkle
### www.anniesprinkle.org

Annie Sprinkle is so many things, including a performance artist, sex educator, porn star, and pioneer. Her website tells her story and provides some of her great writings and musings on things like the G-spot and the seven types of female orgasms. Plus, check out her performance piece about masturbating onstage.

### Barbara Nitke
### www.barbaranitke.com

Barbara's visual images of porn stars and other sexual personae capture the real moments of sex. If you're looking for some visual stimulation, check out Barbara's photography, which you can see on her site.

**Betty Dodson**

**www.bettydodson.com**

Not only should you read her book, but you should buy *all* of her masturbation videos. On her website, you'll find musings on sex and politics, as well as information, advice, and a place to purchase some of Betty's favorite toys, including Betty's Barbell. Every one of Betty's videos is an education, including her latest, *Orgasmic Women: 13 Selfloving Divas,* which shows how thirteen different women jill off.

**Carol Queen**

**www.carolqueen.com**

Carol's the cofounder of the Center for Sex and Culture—the place that sponsors the most famous of all masturbate-a-thons—as well as an award-winning author, a sex educator, and the staff sexologist at Good Vibrations. Check out her recommended reading for a list of all types of sex books.

**Candida Royalle**

**www.candidaroyalle.com**

Famed adult film director Candida Royalle's site allows you to browse her complete catalog of women- and couple-friendly erotica, while also filling you in on the director's life and upcoming projects.

**Clitical.com**

**www.clitical.com**

This site focuses on two of the top sex organs—the clitoris and the mind. With sex tutorials, top-ten lists, erotic stories, and forums to discuss sexuality in the news, Clitical is a great place to visit when you've got sex on the brain.

### Darklady's Masturbate-a-thon
### www.masturbate-a-thon.org

For the past six years, Darklady has made Portland a great place to celebrate the party in your pants. Darklady donates the profits from her masturbate-a-thon parties to organizations that help keep America sex-positive. If you're in or around Portland, Oregon, check out this once-a-year event. And stop by her website for more masturbation resources, including lots of links and articles.

### Ducky DooLittle
### www.duckydoolittle.com

Ducky DooLittle does a lot more than most people will ever do. Once a peep-show girl, burlesque dancer, and dominatrix, Ducky has emerged as one of the nation's top sex educators. Her information is honest, geeky, good clean fun. Easy to read, easy to understand, and well worth checking out. Make sure to peruse her 264 ways to say *vagina* and her tips on exploring erotica.

### Feminists for Free Expression
### www.ffeusa.org

This is a site dedicated to preserving everyone's individual rights with regard to reading, listening, viewing, and producing sexual (and other) materials without government intervention. It's an organization devoted to protecting freedom of expression.

### Feminist Women's Health Center
**www.fwhc.org**

Since 1980, the Feminist Women's Health Center has been promoting and protecting women's rights with regard to reproductive health. They have a section of links to other positive books, places, and resources.

### Femmerotic
**www.femmerotic.com**

This site was founded by Heather Corinna, founder and editor of two other great sex sites, Scarlet Letters and Scarleteen. Her erotic work can be found online and in print all over the place. Her erotic stories webzine *Scarlet Letters* is on hiatus, but check back often, as you never know when things might change. Femmerotic is a subscription site, but if you're looking for more verbal and visual titillation, Ms. Corinna can and will show you the way.

### Fleshbot
**www.fleshbot.com**

An online resource about the newest and freshest things coming out of Porn Valley and beyond, *Fleshbot*'s the web magazine about pornography and the sex culture. It gets updated daily.

### Go Ask Alice!
**www.goaskalice.columbia.edu**

Columbia University's online health service provides answers to myriad questions, from masturbation statistics to STIs (sexually transmitted infections). Offering reliable and accessible information about sexual health/sexuality, this site is a great resource for all your sex-ed questions.

### Jackinworld

**www.jackinworld.com**

Yes, this is a site for male masturbation, but if you want to share the joys of solo sex with your friends/lovers of the opposite sex, direct them here. This sex-positive masturbation site has been online since 1996, and it's great for boys and for girls who like boys!

### Jamye Waxman

**www.jamyewaxman.com**

If you want to learn more about me, here's the place to do it. Check out my podcasts, blog, classes, other writing, and more link recommendations. I'm constantly adding to the site, so stay in touch!

### JanesGuide.com

**www.janesguide.com**

JanesGuide.com reviewers "waste their time so you don't have to." Bringing you cream-of-the-crop listings in their myriad categories (including sexuality resources and erotica), this is the place to go before you start to surf the Net for sexual content. The site's been referred to as the *Consumer Reports* of porn, and honestly, it is.

### Joani Blank

**www.joaniblank.com**

Joani Blank is the woman responsible for lots of sex-positive ventures, including Good Vibrations and Down There Press. She's written and edited tons of stuff on masturbation, from books for children to a book of first-person accounts (*First Person Sexual: Women and Men Write About Self-Pleasuring*, Down There Press, 1996). I love *Femalia* (see the "Required Reading" section) and think Blank is just one groovy, sexy mama.

## Lou Paget

**www.loupaget.com**

Lou Paget is not only a superb sex educator, she is the author of five well-written, factual, and fun sex books, and her advice has been translated into twenty-six languages! Her site isn't chock full of sex information, but you can find out where she's speaking next, watch her on TV, or shop on her site.

## Lusty Lady

**www.lustylady.blogspot.com**

Rachel Kramer Bussel is the lusty lady referred to here, and her blog-spot isn't only the daily musings of a sex-positive vixen, it's also a great place to find hot erotic resources, including Rachel's own books and writings, and other fantastic links.

## Masturbate-a-thon

**www.masturbate-a-thon.com**

This is the link to the San Francisco Masturbate-a-thon, and it's a site that's most active in the month before the actual event in May.

## The Masturbation Interviews

**www.themasturbationinterviews.com**

If you wanna read what other people think about masturbation, this site posts in-depth, and often erotic, interviews with prolific, famous, and influential appreciators—and practitioners—of self-love.

## Masturbation Passion

**www.masturbation-passion.com/en**

The homepage is in French, but if you don't *parlez français*, don't worry. There's a tab for the English version of the site in the top right-hand corner. This is a place for women to share their personal stories, experiences, photos, and confessions about masturbation.

### Nancy Friday
**www.nancyfriday.com**

Nancy Friday's site isn't updated much, but it's a good place to go if you want to check out all seven of her books, take one of her polls, or read some of her insights on sex and beauty.

### Our Bodies, Ourselves
**www.ourbodiesourselves.org**

This is the companion website to the *Our Bodies, Ourselves* books. With supplementary information on anything you can find in the print edition, there's a lot of useful information on the site about women's bodies and our rights.

### Pretty Dumb Things
**www.prettydumbthings.typepad.com**

I really like the long and thoughtful musings of Chelsea Girl, who declares, "Life's too short for both bad grammar and bad sex." She's got great posts on the G-spot and her May 8, 2006, post, "10 pretty dumb things to do when you can't come," is a handy helper. Actually, there are lots of other things to love about Chelsea Girl (mainly her big, big brain)—and she's got lots of great links for your perusing enjoyment.

### Pucker Up
**www.puckerup.com**

Tristan Taormino is super well-known for being the anal queen, and not in that retentive sort of way. On her site you can find sex advice (on butt stuff and other things), as well as her regular *Village Voice* columns and links to her popular *Chemistry* video series (Vivid Videos).

**Regina Lynn**

**www.reginalynn.com/wordpress**

Regina Lynn is the "Sex Drive" columnist at Wired.com, but her personal site allows her to post on a more regular, intimate basis. Here she explores all things sex and tech. For the latest on gadgets and gizmos, and for some great reading, be sure to check her out.

**Scarleteen**

**www.scarleteen.com**

Heather Corinna's site provides feminist sex education for the high school and college crowds, but anyone can, and should, peruse this well-designed site. A writer, activist, sex educator, and advice-giver, Corinna wears all her hats well. You should definitely check out what she's got to say on the subject of masturbation (or anything else, for that matter).

**Seskuality**

**www.seskuality.com**

A website highlighting one woman's exploration of sexuality. Not only does Seska share her personal discoveries, she also takes on sex-themed current events, news, advice, and more. This is a sex-positive site with lots of sex-positive information, including great insights on masturbation.

### SexEdvice

**www.sexedvice.com**

> A lot of people have questions, and Ellen Kate Friedrichs has the answers. A sex educator with a master's in human sexuality education from New York University, Friedrichs's site has a host of her own writing, including articles on masturbation and Betty Dodson.

### Sex Etc.

**www.sexetc.org**

> Sex Etc. is written by teens, for teens. With articles on masturbation, as well as emotional health, relationships, and body image, all teenagers and young adults should click around on this site at least once.

### Sexual Health Network

**www.sexualhealth.com**

> The Sexual Health Network is all about providing access to sexuality information, education, support, and other resources. In their Women's Sexual Health section, you can get information on everything from desire to overstimulation, and the sexual health editorial team is top in the field. With a large focus on disability and sex, this site is one to bookmark.

### Sexuality.org

**www.sexuality.org**

> This site has references, articles, stories, and information on everything sex. It's easy to search for what you're looking for and find a lot of resources. A search for "masturbation" led to lots of outlets.

## Susie Bright
### www.susiebright.blogs.com

Susie Bright edits and writes lots of hot erotica, and her website/blog isn't only intellectually stimulating—it will also keep you in the loop both politically and sexually. Plus, it's a great resource for sexy reading material.

## Tiny Nibbles
### www.tinynibbles.com

This is the web home of Violet Blue, one of the hardest-working women on the web. An intelligent and amazing sex educator, Ms. Blue has written fantastically informative pieces on all things sex, including unsafe sex toys, how to find good porn, and how to surf for porn safely. She's also the editor of lots of hot erotica and other goodies.

## Too Tall Blondes
### www.tootallblondes.com

Barbara Carrellas and Kate Bornstein are the fabulous duo that make up Too Tall Blondes. If you're ever questioning gender, or looking for how to connect better with your own body through breath and other types of orgasms, this is the place to be.

## Viviane's Sex Carnival
### www.thesexcarnival.com

This group blog features erotica, sex news, sexual health information, and cultural posts. It's a great place to start any search for sex on the web.

**Waking Vixen**

**www.wakingvixen.com**

> Audacia Ray is one of the best sex bloggers on the web, and she's got a fabu list of resources for your linking pleasure. Check out her recommendations under Good Smut for some erotic titillation.

**Women's Health News**

**www.womenshealthnews.wordpress.com**

> The informative site is run by a medical librarian out of Nashville, Tennessee. While her focus isn't on masturbation, the blog is a great place for women's health news, information, and other resources.

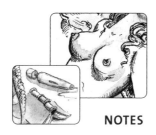

## NOTES

### 1 THE ANATOMY OF ORGASM

1. Rebecca Chalker, *The Clitoral Truth: The Secret World at Your Fingertips* (New York: Seven Stories Press, 2000), 16.

2. Ibid, 87; Mary Jane Sherfey, "The Evolution and Nature of Female Sexuality in Relation to Psychoanalytic Theory," *Journal of the American Psychoanalytic Association* 14, no. 1 (1966).

3. From a phone conversation between Rebecca Chalker and Jamye Waxman, April 24, 2007.

4. Chalker, *The Clitoral Truth*, 16, 36.

5. Ernest Gräfenberg, "The Role of Urethra in Female Orgasm," *International Journal of Sexology*, August 10, 2002, www.doctorg.com/Grafenberg.htm (accessed January 6, 2007).

6. Sexual Health Network "Human Sexual Response Cycles," May 4, 2004, www.sexualhealth.com/article/read/sexuality-education/human-sexual-response-cycles/243 (accessed January 10, 2007).

7. Betty Dodson, *Orgasms for Two: The Joy of Partnersex* (New York: Harmony Books, 2002), 70–77.

8. Lou Paget, *The Big O* (New York: Broadway Books, 2001), 98–112.

9. Barbara Carrellas, *Urban Tantra: Sacred Sex for the Twenty-First Century* (Berkeley: Celestial Arts, 2007), 40, 55–56, 59, 83.

10. Jamye Waxman, "Barbara Carrellas Gives the Skinny on Tantric Sex," Souldish.com, October 17, 2006, www.souldish.com/2006/10/17/barbara-carrellas-gives-the-skinny-on-tantric-sex (accessed January 12, 2007).

11. Annie Sprinkle, *Dr. Sprinkle's Spectacular Sex* (New York: Jeremy P. Tarcher/Penguin, 2005), 262–65.

12. Carrellas, *Urban Tantra*, 83.

## 2 WHAT'S YOUR PLEASURE?

1. Shere Hite, *The Hite Report: A Nationwide Survey on Female Sexuality* (New York: Macmillan, 1976), 5–56.

2. Martha Cornog. *The Big Book of Masturbation: From Angst to Zeal* (San Francisco: Down There Press, 2003), 69.


## 3 THE BUZZ

1. Durex, *Global Sex Survey 2004*, www.durex.com (accessed April 22, 2007).

2. Rachel P. Maines, *The Technology of Orgasm* (Baltimore: Johns Hopkins University Press, 1999), 23.

3. Ibid., 14–15.

4. Ibid., 15–16.

5. Ibid., 100.

6. Ibid., 19–20.

7. Ibid., 105–107.

8. Cynthia Kling, "Love Machines," *Wired*, January 1999, www.wired.com /wired/archive/7.01/vibrators.html (accessed February 12, 2007).

9. Cory Silverberg, "Phthalates in Sex Toys," About.com, March 9, 2007 (accessed April 22, 2007).

10. Violet Blue, "Sex Toy Company Adam and Eve's Official Statement About Sex Toys with Phthalates," Tiny Nibbles, January 31, 2007, www.tinynibbles.com /blogarchives/2007/01/sex_toy_company_adam_and_eves_1.html (accessed February 14, 2007).

11. Jenn Ramsey, "Attack of the Pthalates," *AVN Novelty Business*, January/ February 2007, 38–48.


## 4 SELF-LOVE AND SEX TOYS

1. Michael Hayes, "11th Circuit Court of Appeals Says: No Fundamental Right to Sex Toys," Xbiz.com, February 15, 2007, www.xbiz.com/news_piece (accessed March 3, 2007).

2. Jeff and Kris Booth, "Dildos 101," Erotic University, August 21, 2003, www .eroticuniversity.com/classes/online/dildos.htm (accessed April 22, 2007).

3. Cathy Winks and Anne Semans, *The Good Vibrations Guide to Sex* (San Francisco: Cleis Press, 2002), 183.

4. Keston Huntington, "The History of the Dildo," LezBeOut.com, February 2004, www.lezbeout.com/thehistoryofthedildo_000.htm (accessed April 22, 2007).

5. Winks and Semans, *The Good Vibrations Guide to Sex*, 201.

6. Wikipedia, "Ben Wa balls," http://en.wikipedia.org/wiki/Ben_Wa_balls (accessed April 22, 2007).

7. Maria Burke, "EU Bans Phthalates in Children's Toys," *Environmental Science and Technology Online*, September 7, 2005, http://pubs.acs.org/subscribe/journals/esthag-w/2005/sep/policy/mb_toys.html (accessed February 12, 2007).

8. "Greenpeace Confirms: Topco Sales' CyberSkin Products Phthalate Free," *Business Wire*, September 15, 2006, http://findarticles.com/p/articles/mi_m0EIN/is_2006_Sept_15/ai_n16728383 (accessed April 22, 2007).

9. *The Health Report*, ABC Radio, Australia, March 26, 2007, www.abc.net.au/rn/healthreport (accessed April 22, 2007).

10. Telephone interview between Rachel Venning and Jamye Waxman, December 18, 2006.

11. Durex, *Global Sex Survey 2005*, www.durex.com (accessed April 22, 2007).

## 5  SELF-FULFILLING FANTASIES

1. Robert T. Michael, John H. Gagnon, Edward O. Laumann, and Gina Kolata, *Sex in America: A Definitive Survey* (New York: Little, Brown, 1994), 157.

2. Ibid.

## 6  THE STIGMA OF SOLO SEX

1. Jenne, "Masturbation Madness," Clitical.com, www.clitical.com/female-masturbation/masturbation-madness.php (accessed March 9, 2007).

2. James Carville, *Crossfire*, CNN, December 2, 2004.

3. Jean Stengers and Anne Van Neck, *Masturbation: The History of a Great Terror* (New York: Palgrave, 2001), 9–12, 15–16, 40, 87–88, 104, 143–44.

4. Erika Kinetz, "Is Hysteria Real? Brain Images Say Yes," *The New York Times*, September 26, 2006, www.nytimes.com/2006/09/26/science/26hysteria.html.

5. Laura Briggs, "The Race of Hysteria: Overcivilization and the Savage Woman in Late Nineteenth-Century Obstetrics and Gynecology," *American Quarterly* 52 (2000): 246–73.

6. Kinetz, "Is Hysteria Real?"

7. Beverly Whipple, quoted in *The Health Report*, ABC Radio, Australia, March 26, 2007.

8. Sarah Mahoney, "How Love Keeps You Healthy," *Prevention*, www.prevention .com/article/0,5778,s1-1-83-147-6376-1-P,00.html.

9. Bernadette Condren, "DYO Sexuality for Older Women," *Courier Mail*, March 10, 2007, www.news.com.au/couriermail. Aside from this article, the study "What Does Sexuality Mean to Older Women?" is one of several research projects being done under the banner of the Longitudinal Assessment of Ageing in Women (LAW) at the Royal Brisbane and Women's Hospital's Betty Byrne Henderson Women's Health Research Centre.

10. Joycelyn Elders, *Crossfire*, CNN, April 24, 2001.

11. Condren, "DYO Sexuality for Older Women."

12. Jon Knowles, "Masturbation—from Stigma to Sexual Health," Planned Parenthood Federation of America, November 20, 2002, www.plannedparenthood.org/news-articles-press/politics-policy-issues/ medical-sexual-health/masturbation-6360.htm.

### 7   THE GOOD, THE BAD, AND THE UGLY

1. Giorgi Giorgio and Mario Siccardi, letter to the editor, *American Journal of Obstetrics and Gynecology* 175, no. 3 (1996): 753.

2. Stefan Anitei, "Do Animals Masturbate?" Softpedia, January 12, 2007, http:// news.softpedia.com/news/Do-Animals-Masturbate-44324.shtml.

3. Sharon Gursky, "Sociality in the Spectral Tarsier, Tarsius Spectrum." *American Journal of Primatology* 51 (2000): 89–101.

4. Bruce McFarland, "Masturbation Throughout History,"  www.jackinworld.com /library/articles/history.html.

5. Marguerite Johnson and Terry Ryan, *Sexuality in Greek and Roman Society and Literature: A Sourcebook* (New York: Routledge, 2005), 175–76.

6. Glowka Wayne, "Male and Female Modes of Creation," www.faculty.de.gcsu .edu/~dvess/ids/fap/mfcreat.htm.

7. Thomas W. Laqueur, *Solitary Sex: A Cultural History of Masturbation* (New York: Zone Books, 2003), 112–17.

8. Ibid., 93–94.

9. Stengers and Van Neck, *Masturbation,* 32.

10. Laqueur, *Solitary Sex,* 147.

11. Uta Ranke-Heinemann, *Eunuchs for the Kingdom of Heaven* (New York: Doubleday, 1990).

12. Laqueur, *Solitary Sex,* 161–65.

13. Stengers and Van Neck, *Masturbation,* 37–43.

14. Ibid., 49–50.

15. Richard C. Sha, "Scientific Forms of Sexual Knowledge in Romanticism." *Romanticism on the Net* 23 (August 2001), www.erudit.org/revue/ron/2001/v /n23/005993ar.html.

16. Stengers and Van Neck, *Masturbation,* 74.

17. Ibid., 57–59.

18. Laqueur, *Solitary Sex,* 45.

19. Thomas W. Laqueur, *Making Sex: Body and Gender from the Greeks to Freud* (Cambridge: Harvard Press, 1990), 229.

20. Gale: Free Resources, "Elizabeth Blackwell," 1997, www.gale.com/free_resources /whm/bio/blackwell_e.htm.

21. Laqueur, *Solitary Sex,* 64–66.

22. Thomas Stephen Szasz, *The Manufacture of Madness: A Comparative Study of the Inquisition and the Mental Health Movement* (Syracuse: Syracuse University Press, 1997), 191.

23. Colin Blakemore and Sheila Jennett, *The Oxford Companion to the Body* (Oxford, UK: Oxford University Press, 2001).

24. Carol Groneman, *Nymphomania: A History* (New York: W. W. Norton, 2000), 21.

25. Laqueur, *Solitary Sex,* 363.

26. Groneman, *Nymphomania,* 20–21.

27. John Studd, "Ovariotomy and Menstrual Madness—Lessons for Current Practice," February 19, 2006, www.gynaecology.co.uk/premenstrual syndrome.htm.

28. Blakemore and Jennett, *The Oxford Companion to the Body.*

29. World Health Organization, "Female Genital Mutilation," Fact Sheet No. 241, June 2000, www.who.int/mediacentre/factsheets/fs241/en.

30. Rotten.com, "Kellogg's Cornflakes," April 4, 2003, www.rotten.com/library/sex
    /masturbation/kelloggs-cornflakes.

31. Carrie McLaren, "Porn Flakes: Kellogg, Graham and the Crusade for Moral
    Fiber," *Stay Free!* October 22, 2004, www.stayfreemagazine.org/10
    /graham.htm.

32. Ibid.

33. Cory Silverberg, "Important Events in the History of Masturbation,"
    About.com, May 1, 2006, http://sexuality.about.com/od/masturbation/a
    /masturbationhis.htm.

34. Stengers and Van Neck, *Masturbation*, 133–34.

35. Laqueur, *Solitary Sex*, 367–68.

36. Ibid., 370–72.

37. Groneman, *Nymphomania*, 43.

38. Edward L. Rowan, *The Joy of Self-Pleasuring* (New York: Prometheus, 2000), 124.

39. Laqueur, *Solitary Sex*, 373–74.

40. William H. Masters, Virginia E. Johnson, and Robert C. Kolodny, *Masters and
    Johnson on Sex and Human Loving* (Boston: Little, Brown, 1988), 21.

41. Ibid., 287.

42. Ibid., 21.

43. Jonathan Gathorne-Hardy, *Sex the Measure of All Things: A Life of Alfred C.
    Kinsey* (London: Chatto and Windus, 1998), 395, 399.

44. Alfred C. Kinsey, Wardell B. Pomeroy, Clyde E. Martin, and Paul H. Gebhard,
    *Sexual Behavior in the Human Female* (Philadelphia: W. B. Saunders, 1953),
    142–44.

45. Masters, Johnson, and Kolodny, *Masters and Johnson on Sex and Human
    Loving*, 283.

46. Stengers and Van Neck, *Masturbation*, 168.

47. Rowan, *The Joy of Self-Pleasuring*, 126.

48. Hite, *The Hite Report*, 5–56.

49. Betty Dodson, *Sex for One: The Joy of Selfloving* (New York: Three Rivers
    Press, 1996), 57.

50. Samuel Janus and Cynthia Janus, *The Janus Report on Sexual Behavior* (New York: John Wiley & Sons, 1993).

51. J. Kenneth Davidson and Nelwyn B. Moore, "Masturbation and Premarital Sexual Intercourse Among College Women: Making Choices for Sexual Fulfillment," *Journal of Sex and Marital Therapy* 20, no. 3 (1994): 178–99.

52. Michael et al., *Sex in America*, 158, 165.

53. Leon Panetta, "Press Briefing by Chief of Staff Leon Panetta," White House Office of the Press Secretary, December 9, 1994, www.ibiblio.org/pub /archives/whitehouse-papers/1994/Dec/1994-12-09-Panetta-Briefing-on -Elders-Resignation.

## 8  THE *M* WORD

1. Michael et al., *Sex in America*, 158.

2. Ibid., 162–68.

3. Seska Lee, "Locker Room Sex Talk Part 2," January 17, 2007, www.seskuality.com /article_lockerroom_sextalk.htm.

4. "The World's Largest Collection of Female Masturbation Synonyms," World Wide Wank, October 10, 2002, www.worldwidewank.com/synonyms3.html.

5. Richard Simpson, "Britney Has Sex—Alone," *Evening Standard*, November 13, 2003, www.thisislondon.co.uk/news.

6. Associated Press, "Controversy Sprouts over Prince's Super Bowl Halftime Show," February 7, 2007, www.foxnews.com/story/0,2933,250581,00.html.

7. Tamara Hardingham-Gill, "Celebs and Their Sex Toys," February 7, 2006, www.handbag.com/galleries/gallery/Sex/rels_celebsextoys/MemberID=1/.

8. Erik Hedegaard, "Eva Longoria: A Year of Sex for the Star of *Desperate Housewives*," *Rolling Stone*, December 15, 2004, www.rollingstone.com /poylongoria.

9. "David Beckham's Million-Dollar Sex Toy," SFGate.com, November 12, 2004, www.sfgate.com/cgi-bin/article.cgi?file=/gate/archive/2004/11/12/ ddish.DTL&type=printable.

10. Sharon Krum, "Flying High," *Guardian*, July 17, 2003, www.guardian.co.uk /women/story/0,3604,999556,00.html.

11. Ibid.

12. Wikipedia, http://en.wikipedia.org/wiki/Deenie, December 15, 2005.

13. Judy Blume, February 16, 1998, www.judyblume.com/deenie.html.

14. Wikipedia, http://en.wikipedia.org/wiki/The_Contest, December 6, 2006.

15. Lebby Eyres, "She's Got Bottle," *Bint*, September 8, 2005, www.bintmagazine
.com/bint_stories/906.php?story_id=738.

16. Lester Haines, "Channel 4 to Televise UK's First 'Masturbate-a-thon,'" *Register*,
July 18, 2006, www.theregister.co.uk/2006/07/18/tv_spectacular.

17. Lester Haines, "Channel 4 Pulls 'Wank Week,'" *Register*, February 2, 2007,
www.theregister.co.uk/2007/02/02/channel_four_pulls_series.

18. SIECUS, "Exclusive Purpose: Abstinence-Only Proponents Create Federal
Entitlement in Welfare Reform," December 3, 1998, www.siecus.org/policy
/SReport/srep0001.html.

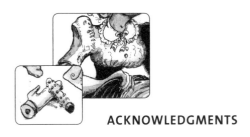

## ACKNOWLEDGMENTS

THIS BOOK WOULDN'T have happened without Audacia Ray, so a million thank-yous to you AR. You are not only a magnificent ally, but also one gem of a friend. I will always be grateful—both to and for you.

Thanks to everyone at Seal, especially my editor Brooke Warner, whose unbiased eyes helped me to not only broaden my own perspectives, but really deconstruct, and reconstruct, the way I talk about sexuality. Thanks also to Laura Mazer, Darcy Cohan and Anne Matthews for their hard work on the book.

Molly Crabapple, how lucky I am to have you illustrating this book. You're such a talented illustrator and I'm very lucky to have worked with you before you got too famous and expensive.

To the woman who started the M revolution—Betty Dodson. Not only are you a fine artist, a top-of-the-line sex educator, a true goddess, and a sexual and artistic pioneer, you are also one of the boldest, most outspoken, honest, funny, and warmhearted women I know. I feel so blessed to know you and I cherish every single second that we get to spend together.

This book couldn't have happened without the women who shared their solo sex lives with me. Thank you for sharing yourselves with me. I appreciate all of you.

That appreciation extends to all the ladies who came to my house in December: Katie, Michelle, Kimb, Lauren, Anu, Cara, Susan, and Yen. Thank you for your candor and for having such interest in this work.

There are so many sex educators who have touched my life, and continue to do so. Candida Royalle, thank you for being my mentor and one of my dearest friends. I not only admire you but feel fortunate to have you on my side. Barbara Carrellas, Joani Blank, Rebecca Chalker, Rachel Venning, Nancy Friday, Annie Sprinkle, Carol Queen, Lou Paget, Ducky DooLittle, Regina Lynn, Violet Blue, Rachel Kramer Bussel, Em and Lo, Anne Semans, Cathy Winks, Abby Ehmann, Kate Bornstein, Cory Silverberg, Seska, and all the other sex educators who helped me with this project, either knowingly or unbeknownst to them (that would be a big thank-you to everyone whose work I've ever flipped through or whom I've ever had the pleasure of learning anything from).

Babeland, and Claire Cavanah, you gave me an experience that money can't buy.

To *Playgirl*. You are not only a place where a girl can read about fantasies, but for me you have made my fantasy of being a sex advice columnist come true.

To Circe. You are a gifted photographer, and I'm so lucky to have been "captured" by you.

To the board of Feminists for Free Expression. Thank you for taking me under your wings and supporting me. I am grateful to walk among such an extraordinary group of women.

Cousin Robin, thank you for stepping up to the plate and providing me with your time, love, and expertise when I needed your help. You are great family.

To Leslie, Amy, Susanna, Catherine, Stacey, Heather, Mischa, and Marybeth, for shining your goddess light on me all the time. Extra-special thanks to Amy for rocking so hard during crunch time.

The support of my family is amazing. You love and accept me for who I am and who I've become. Thank you for being proud of me and loving me, no matter what.

Blue. You remind me that sleep, food, and cuddling on the couch every so often are all part of the necessities of life.

Jonny. Thanks for not only loving me and editing my work, but for putting up with my jazz hands. I never thought I'd be so lucky as to meet someone as kind, caring, and compassionate as you are. You are my partner, and friend, and I love you more and more all the time.

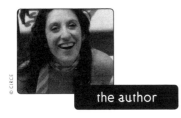

**the author**

JAMYE WAXMAN has been dubbed "the nexxxt generation of sex educator" by Wired.com. She has her master's in sex ed from Widener University, and is the sex advice columnist for *Playgirl*; her work also appears in *Women's Health, Men's Health, Zink, Steppin' Out,* and the *Philly Edge.* Jamye contributed to the book *Naked Ambition: Women Who Are Changing Pornography* (Carroll and Graf). She is creator, director, and host of the *Personal Touch* video series for Adam and Eve Pictures. She knows about vibrators, dildos, and butt plugs, thanks to her five years working at the world-famous sex shop Babeland in NYC. Jamye serves as president of Feminists for Free Expression and lives in Brooklyn, New York. You can find her blog (one of About.com's favorite sex blogs of 2006) and podcasts at www.jamyewaxman.com.

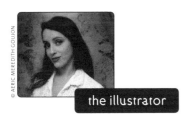

**the illustrator**

MOLLY CRABAPPLE is an artist known for her surreal, sexy Victoriana. She's wielded her pen for clients like *The New York Times, The Wall Street Journal,* Marvel Comics, and *Playgirl,* while hanging her work in galleries across America. Her first book, *Dr. Sketchy's Official Rainy Day Colouring Book,* was released in 2006. She lives in Brooklyn, New York.

# SELECTED TITLES FROM SEAL PRESS

*For more than thirty years, Seal Press has published groundbreaking books.*

*By women. For women.*

*Visit our website at* **www.sealpress.com**.

*Indecent: How I Make It and Fake It as a Girl for Hire* by Sarah Katherine Lewis. $14.95, 1-58005-169-3. An insider reveals the gritty reality behind the alluring facade of the sex industry.

*Single State of the Union: Single Women Speak Out on Life, Love, and the Pursuit of Happiness* edited by Diane Mapes. $14.95, 1-58005-202-9. Written by an impressive roster of single (and some formerly single) women, this collection portrays single women as individuals whose lives extend well beyond Match.com and Manolo Blahniks.

*Confessions of a Naughty Mommy: How I Found My Lost Libido* by Heidi Raykeil. $14.95, 1-58005-157-X. The Naughty Mommy shares her bedroom woes and woo-hoos with other mamas who are rediscovering their sex lives after baby and are ready to think about it, talk about it, and *do* it.

*Inappropriate Random: Stories on Sex and Love* edited by Amy Prior. $13.95, 1-58005-099-9. This collection of short fiction by women writers takes a hard look at love today—exposing its flaws with unflinching, often hilarious candor.

*Unruly Appetites: Erotic Stories* by Hanne Blank. $14.95, 1-58005-081-6. Erotic fiction with sensual lyricism and dynamic characters that titillate and inspire.

*Shameless: Women's Intimate Erotica* edited by Hanne Blank. $14.95, 1-58005-060-3. Diverse and delicious memoir-style erotica by today's hottest fiction writers.